ABOUT THE AUTHOR

Maryon Stewart studied preventive dentistry and nutrition at the Royal Dental Hospital in London and worked as a counsellor with nutritional doctors in England for four years. At the beginning of 1984 she set up the PMT Advisory Service which has subsequently helped thousands of women worldwide. In 1987 she launched the Women's Nutritional Advisory Service which now provides broader help to women of all ages.

Maryon Stewart is the author of the best-selling books *No More PMS!* (formerly *Beat PMS Through Diet*), now in its third edition, *Beat Sugar Craving*, *Beat the Menopause without HRT*, *Healthy Parents, Healthy Baby* and *Every Woman's Health Guide*. She is the co-author of *The Vitality Diet*, *No More IBS!*, *The PMS Cookbook* and *Every Woman's Health Guide*. She has her own weekly radio programme on health and nutrition, has co-written several medical papers and has written articles for many magazines including *Marie Claire, Cosmopolitan, Chat, Woman's Journal*, BBC *Good Health, Woman's Own, Health & Fitness* and for both the *Daily Mirror* and the *Daily Mail*.

She has also appeared on several popular TV magazine shows, such as TV AM, GMTV, Top of the Morning, Channel Four Food File, BBC Here & Now, Good Morning with Anne & Nick, Reportage, Meridian, Carlton, MSkyB, The Miriam Stoppard Health & Beauty Show, This Morning, Pebble Mill, Channel Four, Streetwise and TVS. She has contributed regularly to Capital Woman, has done a series of programmes for Yorkshire TV's 'Help Yourself' programmes and has helped Anglia TV with the 'Bodyworks' series.

Maryon has written her own regular page in the magazines *House and Garden* and *Healthy Eating*, and now is both advisor and contributor to *Good Health* magazine. She is on the Panel of Advisors for First Steps Magazine and frequently lectures to both the lay public and the medical profession. She is married to Dr Alan Stewart and they live in Lewes, Sussex, with their four children.

'No illness which can be treated by diet should be treated by any other means.'

Maimonides, twelfth-century physician

Other titles by Maryon Stewart and Dr Alan Stewart

Beat Sugar Craving by Maryon Stewart
The Vitality Diet by Maryon Stewart and Dr Alan Stewart
Nutritional Medicine by Dr Stephen Davies and Dr Alan Stewart
Tired all the Time by Dr Alan Stewart
Beat PMS Cookbook by Maryon Stewart and Sarah Tooley
No More IBS! by Maryon Stewart and Dr Alan Stewart
Beat the Menopause without HRT by Maryon Stewart
Healthy Parents, Healthy Baby by Maryon Stewart
Every Woman's Health Guide by Maryon Stewart and Dr Alan Stewart

NO MORE PMS!

*The medically proven Women's
Nutritional Advisory Service Programme*

Maryon Stewart

with contributions from
Dr Alan Stewart

Vermilion
LONDON

To Sue Fisher Hendry – who has earned her stripes as a sister and a valid friend

IMPORTANT NOTE FOR SUFFERERS

There are many fairly technical terms used to describe the Pre-Menstrual Syndrome and the normal menstrual cycle. You may already be familiar with some of the more technical terms, whilst others will be new to you. I have prepared a brief Dictionary of Terms to refer to which begins on page 269. Please don't be afraid to use it as often as necessary. The better you understand the information, the more you will be able to apply it to your own life and symptoms.

If your symptoms occur at other times of the month, apart from during your pre-menstrual time, you should have a medical check-up with your own doctor. If your symptoms are very severe it would be advisable to have your nutritional programme supervised by your own doctor or a trained counsellor. If you get confused or need extra advice, the Women's Nutritional Advisory Service is there to help you. All letters receive a personal reply: their address is on page 301.

This revised edition first published in 1997

19

Text copyright © 1987, 1990, 1994 and 1997 by Maryon Stewart, Dr Guy Abraham

The moral right of Maryon Stewart has been asserted in accordance with the Copyright, Designs and Patents Act, 1988.

First published in the United Kingdom in 1987 by Century Publishing Co. Ltd

This edition published in 1997 by Vermilion
an imprint of Ebury Press
Random House, 20 Vauxhall Bridge Road, London SW1V 2SA

The Random House Group Limited Reg. No. 954009
www.randomhouse.co.uk

A CIP catalogue record for this book
is available from the British Library

ISBN 9780091816223

Illustrations by Mike Gordon

Penguin Random House is committed to a sustainable future for our business, our readers and our planet. This book is made from Forest Stewardship Council® certified paper.

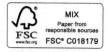

Printed and bound in Great Britain by Clays Ltd, St Ives plc

Typeset by SX Composing, Rayleigh, Essex

CONTENTS

Foreword by Leslie Kenton   vii

Introduction   x

PART ONE   THE REALITIES OF PMS

Chapter 1   A problem as old as the hills   1

Chapter 2   Functioning normally   5

Chapter 3   PMS defined   12

Chapter 4   The making of PMS   15

Chapter 5   Anxious, irritable and uptight   19

Chapter 6   Bloating, weight gain and breast tenderness   37

Chapter 7   Sugar cravings, headaches and fatigue   47

Chapter 8   Depression, crying and thoughts of suicide   57

Chapter 9   Other symptoms – clumsiness, loss of sex drive
and agoraphobia   69

Chapter 10   The social implications of PMS   80

PART TWO   NUTRITION AND OUR BODIES

Chapter 11   Why is PMS more common today?   95

Chapter 12   Medical treatments   113

Chapter 13   Nutritional treatments   120

Chapter 14   Nutrition and the body: vitamins and minerals,
what they do   125

PART THREE   THE NUTRITIONAL APPROACH – A SELF-HELP MANUAL

Chapter 15   Choosing a nutritional plan   147

Chapter 16   A tailor-made nutritional programme – Option 3   164

Chapter 17   Nutritious recipes   208

Chapter 18   Stress or distress?   229

Chapter 19   The value of exercise and relaxation   233

Chapter 20   Other valuable therapies   244

Chapter 21   Other related problems   249

Chapter 22   Men who no longer suffer   263

PART FOUR   APPENDICES

1 Dictionary of terms 269   2 Food additives 272

3 Nutritional supplement suppliers 273   4 Recommended reading list 274

5 Useful addresses 276   6 Charts and diaries 281   7 References 285

Index 291   Further help 301

ACKNOWLEDGEMENTS

I would first like to acknowledge the researchers that have gone before us who collectively completed the groundwork that allowed us to begin our work from an advanced point. In particular I refer to early work by Dr Katharina Dalton, Dr Michael Brush, Dr David Horrobin, Dr Guy Abraham and Professor Shaughn O'Brien.

Special thanks are due to both Dr Alan Stewart and Dr Guy Abraham for their advice and support over the years. Without their technical support we would not have been able to provide such valuable help to so many women, and education on the nutritional approach to Pre-Menstrual Syndrome to so many doctors, nurses and medical organizations.

My heartfelt thanks also go to all the wonderful new patients who have volunteered to share their case histories with us in this book. Their willingness to divulge intimate details so frankly in an effort to help others is highly appreciated.

Next I must thank the caring team that have worked at the Women's Nutritional Advisory Service, in particular Cheryl Griffiths for her organisational skills and her ability to keep calm in a crisis, Helen Heap for battling with our patient records to produce meaningful statistics and Allison Day for her help with research and typing. Without all those acknowledged this book would not have been possible.

I would also like to thank the following people for advice: Deryn Bell on osteopathy, Paul Lundberg on acupuncture and acupressure and Julia Swift on exercise.

Thanks are also due to Lavinia Trevor for her support and the benefit of her wisdom and to Rowena Webb and Anabel Briggs at Vermilion for their enthusiasm and professionalism.

Lastly, I must thank our wonderful nanny, Joanna John, for happily occupying the children whilst I put the third edition of this book together, and the children themselves, Phoebe, Chesney, Hester and Simeon, for unselfishly allowing me time out, and providing me with regular refreshments and cuddles.

Maryon Stewart

FOREWORD
BY
LESLIE KENTON

This is an extraordinary book. Not only does it tackle the very complex subject of Pre-Menstrual Syndrome (PMS) in a simple and straightforward way so that it becomes understandable to the average woman suffering from it, but it is also eminently practical. It tells you exactly how to go about finding the answer to your own difficulties.

PMS, with its symptoms of bloating, depression, irritability, fatigue and all the rest is not something 'normal' which you have to suffer from, month in month out. I have seen even the most resistant cases turn around through changes of diet, alterations in living habits and the judicious use of certain nutritional supplements. What Maryon Stewart has done so cleverly is to explain how to help yourself: first by making you aware of what your specific problems are, and then by helping you outline a self-directed lifestyle programme for solving them.

And Maryon Stewart can substantiate her claims too. Having already put into practice the natural approach to PMS set out in this book for 14 years, and having monitored its results on a thousand women through the Women's Nutritional Advisory Service, she knows what she is talking about. The methods work. And her advice about eating natural organically-grown foods, using simple techniques which can help you better manage stress, calling on well-planned nutritional supplements when necessary and even making use of natural treatments which you can carry out yourself to cope with acute problems is not only sound in relation to eliminating PMS. It can also be taken far beyond to form the basis of a total lifestyle for optimum health for women and men alike. *No More PMS!* is a book to be read, used and then loaned to friends when they need it.

" Claire's Story " *

Claire is a housewife of 36 with two school-aged children and a toddler of 22 months. She suffered with severe PMS for 11 years and described herself as a Jekyll and Hyde character because of her severe mood swings.

'I had suffered for 11 years with a variety of severe symptoms, feeling awful for three weeks out of four. I had totally unpredictable mood swings; I would put my coat on to go to the supermarket, but by the time I reached the front door I couldn't go. I would be submerged in a deep black cloud. I physically attacked my partner, often hitting or punching him. I was venomous and unreasonable. He was so sympathetic at the time which made me feel ashamed of the way I had treated him. I took little interest in sex which was very unlike me. Before I started having problems with PMS it would not be unusual for me to have sex four to six times a week. Now it was just a duty.

I became snappy, short tempered and spiteful with my children. Like Jekyll and Hyde I was very aggressive towards them pre-menstrually, but a normal loving mother once my period had begun. I couldn't plan any day's outing such as swimming or the cinema when I knew I would be pre-menstrual. The children always knew when I wasn't myself as I would be so critical of them. I would be totally unreasonable, shouting at them for the silliest of things. They now tell me that they were afraid of me and thought I was temporarily insane, a mad woman.

I haven't worked since the birth of my first daughter 11 years ago. My son, now 15, became disabled at 4 years old. Later, I did think about returning to work but I couldn't have held a job down with my health being so unpredictable. I struggled with the housework, just hoovering was a major task, and my partner usually took over with the shopping and cleaning to ease the strain. My self esteem was non-existent. I detested myself for not being able to give my children a secure family life. There were many times I didn't want to go on living.

PMS took away all normal life. There was no routine to our existence. I would try hard to get up from bed to send my kids out to school early, but in the morning I would be late and they had to rush to get to school without

* Despite the fact that most of the patients who volunteered to tell their story in the book didn't object to my using their actual names, I felt it would be more appropriate to change their names and let them remain anonymous. They are all real women who have recently overcome their symptoms and were willing to be interviewed.

their breakfast. My parents and partner realised it was an illness and were very supportive. It took all my confidence away and I became just an empty shell. I had tried the contraceptive pill with no success. Ponstan helped with the cramps I would get, temporarily, and I also took anti-depressants which didn't work either. I was desperate.

New diet

I read about the WNAS in a magazine but it took me two years to summon up the courage to make contact with them. They put me on their programme and told me to eat lots of vegetables and fresh fruit, and have plenty of fresh fish. I had to cut out chocolate, caffeine and wheat. At first it was very difficult, but now it's just part of every day life. I also was to take supplements of Efamol, Optivite and Normoglycaemia to control the cravings. It only took about four to five weeks before I was feeling substantially better, and every month I improved greatly, so much so that the symptoms were disappearing and I was feeling my old self once more.

End result

I now feel really well and I'm enjoying life again, am much more energetic and both my skin and nails are healthy. Before, when I was out I would avoid everyone because I was so confused I would struggle to make sense of their words. I go out now with family and friends without any second thought, and the children are much happier with me and we talk about their problems and interests. My partner and I have regained respect and trust for one another again. During the years when I was suffering he found comfort in gambling as he was so unhappy. He now realises why he used to gamble: it was because he wasn't in control of his life with me being ill, and this gave him a false sense of control and security. We have a good sex life once again and thankfully I don't think of it as a need or a duty but as a loving and intimate experience to share.

I now look after the children and my home life and driving is fine all month. There are times when life is stressful, particularly with my son's disability, but I know if I take time to plan and relax and remember how far I've come, I can enjoy my life.'

INTRODUCTION

NO MORE PMS!

When I set out to write my first book on Pre-Menstrual Syndrome in 1986 there was little else available on the bookshelves for the public on this subject. Today, however, it is a pretty crowded marketplace, which begs the question, why did I need to write again on this subject?

Through our efforts at the Women's Nutritional Advisory Service (WNAS) over the last 14 years, we have helped literally tens of thousands of women over their symptoms of PMS. The treatment approach that we have pioneered has become more and more effective as time has passed by. We have now reached the point, where with my hand on my heart, I can honestly say that for the vast majority of women there is no longer any need to suffer with Pre-Menstrual Syndrome. Each year or two we make an assessment of our clinical results and we now know, from repeated studies, that between 90 to 95 per cent of women (depending on the study) are completely over their symptoms within four months.

This new book on PMS is true to its new title *No More PMS!*. It contains the solutions to overcoming all aspects of PMS, and is based on the successful WNAS programme which is currently being used by women all over the world. The programme, which is based on published medical facts, and specifically addresses the causes of PMS, consists of:

- Making dietary changes

- Taking scientifically based nutritional supplements that have been through properly conducted clinical trials, and

- Taking moderate exercise on a regular basis.

THE SECRET LIES IN THE REAL CAUSE OF PMS

To this day, arguments about the cause of PMS between the medical profession persist. While some vehemently believe that the symptoms are caused by a hormone imbalance, others argue that it is a psychological condition: in other words, it is all in the mind. Our research shows that while a bit of both theories have a part to play in the symptoms of PMS, the underlying cause is much more fundamental. Sadly PMS does not have the physical characteristics of an abscess or an ingrown toenail. Neither does it show up under a microscope like a diseased cell. The agony and the anguish suffered, not to mention the misery and the mental torture, cannot easily be measured.

Perhaps because PMS is relatively difficult to detect or quantify by an outsider the condition has taken far longer than it should have done to become recognised, and still longer to be treated effectively without the use of drugs. As a result, women have had to go on suffering unnecessarily. We discovered many years ago that many PMS sufferers have nutritional deficiencies, which disturb both brain chemical metabolism and hormone function; which when corrected restore normal balance in the body so that symptoms disappear.

From the studies we have conducted we have established that of women with PMS, between 50 to 80 per cent (again depending on the study) have low levels of a very important mineral called magnesium. This elevates magnesium into the position of being the most commonly deficient nutrient in women with PMS. Apart from other functions in the body, magnesium is necessary for normal brain chemical metabolism, and the brain chemistry may be compared to the equivalent of a conductor in an orchestra in that it is responsible for orchestrating the workings of the body. Magnesium is also responsible for normal hormone function and for smooth muscle control – and both the gut and the uterus are smooth muscles. When a deficiency of magnesium exists it is likely that both physical and psychological symptoms arrive on the scene, plus it also contributes to bowel disorders like diarrhoea and constipation and to painful periods. That is a large responsibility for a single nutrient.

Additionally, other nutrients may be in short supply. Iron levels are low in approximately 25 per cent of women of child-bearing age, B vitamins are often in short supply too, and sometimes levels of other important nutrients such as zinc and essential fatty acids may also be lacking.

Although many young women suffer with PMS in their teens and early 20s, the majority of women who contact us for help have had one or more children. Many of them only experienced mild PMS symptoms, if any, prior to having their children, which fits in with our theory about nutritional deficiencies. During pregnancy the nutrient demands placed upon a woman's body are far greater that at other times in her life; except for while breastfeeding, when the demands are greater still.

HOW DOES THE WNAS PROGRAMME WORK?

The WNAS programme aims to redress the balance by putting the nutrients back into the body that time and nature have taken out. Restoring the correct nutrient balance in the body has a normalising effect on both brain chemistry and hormone levels; and within a four-month period most symptoms disappear. It's a bit like turning the factory lights back on again!

Unfortunately, our programme does not provide an overnight solution; instead it takes several months to see the full results. Many women, however, do experience considerable relief within the first few months, but there are some who wait three or four months before experiencing relief. The research definitely shows that it can take four months to influence both brain chemistry and hormone levels, so an element of patience and determination is required. Having a supportive partner, family member or friend will aid your progress, and so too will sharing the stories of some of our wonderful case histories, who have been willing to 'tell all' in this book in the hope that they can help others in return for the help that they themselves received from the WNAS.

WHY AREN'T DOCTORS PROVIDING THE SOLUTION?

You may well ask the question 'Why hasn't my doctor provided me with the solution if it is based on published medical science?' Sadly, the answer is that the medical profession, at this time, are lacking knowledge about nutrition, even though the subject of nutrition was taught to undergraduate doctors at the beginning of the twentieth century. According to a WNAS survey on 1,000 general practitioners, 92 per cent admitted having no nutritional training whatsoever on the subject of PMS, despite the fact that most experts now agree that the nutritional approach to PMS is the best first-line treatment. In our survey, 79 per cent of the doctors said that they would like to be educated, but the disappointing fact is that there is currently no facility to bring this about. By doctors' own admission, the average time spent on lectures on nutrition in general during their whole training is between two to four hours, as evidenced by a report in the Journal of the Royal Society of Medicine, that 98 per cent of undergraduates had failed their nutrition paper.

So it comes as no surprise that despite the willingness of most doctors, they are not equipped to give effective advice about conditions such as PMS at this time. There are exceptions, of course, but for the most part the published medical papers on the subject of PMS are behind the doors of the post-graduate medical library, in a variety of medical journals, which makes it exceedingly difficult for a busy doctor to access them.

As a result of the lack of education of doctors, PMS sufferers are often left feeling frustrated and even more depressed as they are left to fend for themselves. We hear all sorts of stories from sufferers who have visited their doctor for advice, which could be considered to be amusing were it not for the fact that these poor women were left suffering. I'll share a few of the comments in the hope that you can see the funny side of them!

When I was nineteen and single my doctor suggested I have a baby in order to overcome my PMS. When I asked him what I should do with the baby once it was born, he slammed his fist on his desk and said, 'You women are all the same. We give you advice and you refuse to take it!' and with that he went to the door and indicated that it was time for me to leave.

As a solution to my PMS my doctor suggested that I join the Conservative Party and become a magistrate, as his wife had done.

My doctor told me that my PMS was a sign that I was rejecting my femininity.

I was told by my doctor that my PMS was all in my mind. But as I gain 12 cm (5 in) pre-menstrually around my middle, I told him indignantly that if it was anywhere it was all in my waist!

'All part of being a woman' is a hot favourite.

To a non-sufferer these tales may sound amusing, but to a woman suffering with PMS who is feeling wretched, and in some cases suicidal, being fobbed off and left to battle with her disrupted existence for up to half of every month that she breathes air, is really no laughing matter.

The WNAS does provide an information service for members of the medical profession, and continues to provide research material in an attempt to spread the word, but realistically this is a mere drop in the ocean of work that needs to be done. You will find one of our recent studies threaded through the first part of the book. This is a study on 500 of the women we have treated recently, looking at the degree of personal suffering that PMS brings and the effect that it has on relationships, the family, the ability to work and interaction with others. This is a repeat of a study we conducted in 1985 on 1,000 patients, and the sad fact is that the statistics are even worse now than they were then, with an increase of 11 per cent of PMS sufferers contemplating suicide pre-menstrually and an additional 3 per cent attempting suicide.

The ideal situation is that the nutritional approach to PMS becomes recognised widely as a valid part of orthodox medicine and is taught to both qualified doctors and those currently studying. In the meantime, this book, which is based on 14 years research and clinical experience at the WNAS, will provide you with the information you need in order to overcome your symptoms. All our advice is based on published medical papers which are referenced at the end of the book for the technically minded.

No More PMS! will explain how you can solve the problem for yourself, according to your own individual symptoms. It is written in four parts.

Part One deals with the realities of Pre-Menstrual Syndrome and the effect it has on both the individual and family life.

Part Two covers nutrition in relation to your body.

Part Three is devoted to diet and other means of self-help and finally, in Part Four you will find lists of useful information and addresses.

While the book is a comprehensive self-help guide, it is not uncommon for women suffering severely with PMS to feel overwhelmed by their symptoms and thus unable to help themselves initially. We also provide clinic services for individuals and a telephone and postal consultation service for those who live too far from the clinics, which is used by women all over the world. You will find the details of how to obtain our help on page 301.

By reading this book you will receive the education that you have missed to date. It will help you over your PMS symptoms in the short term, but additionally will help to improve the quality of both your health and that of your family for many years to come.

Good luck.

PART ONE

THE REALITIES OF PMS

1

A PROBLEM
AS OLD AS
THE HILLS

Despite the fact that for the last few years we have been talking and writing about the Pre-Menstrual Syndrome (PMS) as if it has just been discovered, in reality it has been affecting women all over the world for many years.

I am often asked the question 'How come PMS is more common now than it was years ago?' My answer is that we talk about the condition far more now than we used to, and that there are many aspects relating to the twentieth-century diet and environment that seem to contribute significantly to the problem.

The whole event has become affectionately nicknamed 'The Curse'. It seems that this term derives from ancient times when a menstruating woman was considered by society to be unclean, and in some cases dangerous. In some primitive tribes menstrual blood was considered to be evil, and a menstruating woman had to remain shut away for fear that she would cast a spell on the menfolk or kill off whole herds of animals using her temporary 'witch's' powers. If a menstruating woman disobeyed this or similar rules and mixed with the menfolk, some tribes would even condemn her to death.

Certain religions still regard a menstruating woman as undesirable. In the Moslem religion a menstruating woman is not allowed to enter the mosque. As recently as the beginning of this century a Greek Orthodox woman was not permitted Communion during her period, and to this day in the Orthodox Jewish religion, menstruating women are not permitted to sleep with their husbands during their period.

Is it any wonder that complexes about the whole subject developed and that the subject became taboo? Who, with any degree of sanity, would have wanted to admit the fact that their period was due? It makes the mind boggle!

Despite the fact that women's often frenzied accounts of their unbearable pre-menstrual symptoms have been labelled as being 'all in the mind', i.e. a mental condition, past treatments included hysterectomies, electric shock treatment, and even, in tragic cases, lobotomies (an operation where part of the brain is removed). Traditionally Western medicine tends to regard a physical condition as one that we have no control over and that needs treatment by physical means using drugs and suchlike, and a mental condition as one where the person's personality contributes to the illness. This division is seen as being increasingly artificial.

The first recorded cases of PMS (or PMT, as it was then known) were in 1931, when Dr Robert T. Frank, an American physician working in New York reported 15 cases of Pre-Menstrual Tension. These women had symptoms of nervous tension, water retention and weight gain. Dr Frank found a high level of the hormone oestrogen present in these patients and felt that they were unable to excrete the oestrogen from their bodies premenstrually. The excess oestrogen, he felt, then irritated the nervous system, and thus symptoms developed.

Further work was done by other American doctors in this field. In 1938 Dr Israel, another American doctor, presented his theory that not all women had high levels of oestrogen, but they did have low levels of the hormone progesterone.

In 1943 Dr Biskind published a study which supported the theory that many pre-menstrual symptoms reported were similar to vitamin B deficiency symptoms. He found that treatment with vitamin B greatly improved symptoms, especially uncomfortable breast symptoms and heavy bleeding during menstruation, which are also symptoms of vitamin B deficiency. The cause was an overload of oestrogen pre-menstrually.

As early as 1944 Dr Harris observed women with pre-menstrual fatigue, nervousness and cravings for sweet foods. Further research along these lines continued in the 1950s.

The first scientific publication from the United Kingdom was in 1937 from a group of women doctors led by Dr McCance from King's College Hospital in London. Their detailed survey of 169 mainly professional women documented the presence of increased fatigue, headaches and mood swings occurring pre-menstrually and during the period. These doctors were uncertain as to the exact cause of these physical and mood changes. In 1953 Dr Katharina Dalton, a British doctor, began publishing her work. She and Dr Raymond Greene renamed the condition 'Pre-Menstrual Syndrome', as they identified so many symptoms as being pre-menstrual. Dr Dalton is considered a pioneer in this field. She spent many years identifying the magnitude of the problem in prisons, hospitals, factories, offices and schools. She also studied the relationship between pre-menstrual symptoms and crime, alcoholism and drug abuse. Quite a few of her studies are mentioned later on in the text, as they served as a starting point for our own research. Dr Dalton supports the theory that pre-menstrually low levels of the hormone progesterone are present. Her treatment consists largely of progesterone supplementation.

During the 1970s and 80s there were many attempts to identify a hormonal abnormality – a deficiency in women with PMS when compared with those who did not suffer. Many minor abnormalities, including elevated or decreased levels of progesterone, oestrogen and other hormones, were described in numerous small studies. However, no consistent pattern has emerged and the considered medical wisdom is that the vast majority of sufferers do not have a hormone excess or lack but are perhaps unduly sensitive to the normal swings in hormone levels that occur throughout the menstrual cycle. To support this new concept there is some very good evidence that the most powerful hormonal treatments are highly effective in controlling PMS. The reason for this is that if you can switch off the ovaries then you lose the normal rise and fall of hormone production, abolish the menstrual cycle, cease having periods and thus prevent PMS. No ovaries equals no PMS. Of course you then have a whole host of other problems as a result of this type of treatment.

Other workers have tried to link different patterns of pre-menstrual symptoms with changes either in hormones or in body chemistry. Dr Guy Abraham, a leading researcher from the United States, has over the last 20 years looked in detail at the relationship between nutritional factors, hormone function and PMS. Certain patterns can sometimes be discerned, thus allowing a more rational use of dietary treatments, and sometimes drug or hormonal treatments.

These are covered in some detail later on and we also show the benefits we have obtained using a nutritional approach.

As a group we haven't set out to prove whether it is in fact a physical or mental condition. *We know it is a real condition*. Instead, we approach it from the viewpoint that certain symptoms exist which may be overcome by making dietary changes and adjustments in lifestyles where necessary. Between us we have many years of experience and have been able to help tens of thousands of women around the world to overcome their pre-menstrual problems.

I aim to give you a good understanding of what happens to your body during your monthly cycle. I will then help you to identify what the symptoms may be due to and then, of course, how you can go about getting them sorted out.

2

FUNCTIONING
NORMALLY

THE NORMAL MENSTRUAL CYCLE

In order to understand what is going wrong with your menstrual cycle, it is important to have a fairly good understanding of what the normal menstrual cycle is.

The age at the onset of periods has been decreasing at a rate of three years per century. Periods begin between the tenth and sixteenth year in 95 per cent of European girls, and between the tenth and fifteenth year in American girls. The age at the onset of the menopause, when periods cease, has been increasing at a rate of three years per century as well. Menopause occurs between the ages of 40 and 55.

The menstrual cycle is a fertility cycle, a fascinating process that enables a woman to conceive a child. This cycle is repeated each month, and if fertilization does not occur the cycle ends with a menstrual period – the shedding of the lining of the womb in preparation for the next cycle. The cycle can vary in length from approximately 22 days up to 34 days. Anything between these numbers would be considered normal. The first day of bleeding, the day the period arrives, is referred to as the first day of the cycle.

THE ORGANS INVOLVED

There are specific organs which each play an important role in the menstrual cycle. They are designed to work together so that a woman can become pregnant and nourish the growing child throughout the nine months of pregnancy.

The uterus or womb, as it is more commonly known, is a hollow, pear-shaped muscular organ which is about three inches (7.5 cm) long in a non-pregnant woman. There are many layers of specialized muscle here which, as if by magic, can expand so that the uterus becomes many times its usual size during pregnancy. The growing child lives in the uterus until it is ready to be born.

The innermost layer of the uterus is a membrane called the endometrium. During the cycle it becomes filled with the blood supply which would be needed to nourish a pregnancy. If conception has not occurred the endometrium breaks down, and together with the blood leaves the uterus through the neck of the uterus, which is known as the cervix.

The cervix or neck of the womb is like a little ball towards the back of the vagina. It has a small opening which remains closed for most of the time. A few days before the egg is released by the ovary, the cervix begins to open. By the time the egg has left the ovary, the opening would have become wide enough to let the sperm swim up through it, in order to gain access to the egg.

For a few days each cycle, at the time of ovulation, the specialized cells in the cervix produce fertile cervical mucus, which allows the sperm to live during their journey to the uterus. At other times during the menstrual cycle the cervix produces infertile cervical mucus which prevents the sperm from surviving.

Once the menstrual blood passes through the cervix it flows into the vaginal canal, a four- to six-inch (10–15 cm) muscular tube which has the ability to widen during sexual intercourse and during labour. During intercourse the lining of the vaginal canal becomes engorged with blood. A slippery liquid is produced which is designed to make the experience of sexual intercourse more comfortable.

The two almond-shaped organs on either side of the uterus are called the ovaries. They contain thousands of immature eggs which are present in a baby girl even before birth! From puberty, usually, one egg will leave one ovary during each menstrual cycle. I say usually, as there are occasions when more than one egg becomes fertilized simultaneously, and multiple births result.

OVULATION

The process of the egg leaving the ovary is called ovulation. At about 12 to 16 days before menstruation, the ovary will release an egg. The egg is then usually picked up by one of the Fallopian tubes, which is where the egg and the sperm would meet if conception were to take place. The Fallopian tubes are a pair of very thin tubes, about four inches (10 cm) long, which are connected to each side of the uterus. The egg waits for the sperm in the Fallopian tube for between 12 and 24 hours. If no sperm arrive, the egg is then absorbed by the body. If the egg and the sperm do meet and join up, fertilization takes place, and the fertilized egg will then move down, over the next few days, into the uterus, where it becomes embedded in the lining. This fertilized egg then grows into a baby.

WHAT CONTROLS THE CYCLE?

It is important to understand that although we have looked at the various organs at work for us during the menstrual cycle, it is actually the brain that controls the ovaries. In fact, a particular part of the brain called the pituitary gland sends instructions to the ovaries to make them function. The pituitary gland will tell the ovaries when to produce eggs and release them. It also stimulates production by the ovaries of oestrogen and progesterone, two very special sex hormones. If no fertilization occurs, the pituitary gland will send a new signal for the ovaries to begin producing eggs again.

WHAT ACTUALLY HAPPENS DURING THE CYCLE?

Either just prior to your period arriving, or during your period, several eggs will begin to grow in the ovary. Each egg is surrounded by a sac which is called a follicle. The egg and the follicle grow together. The follicle produces oestrogen which, as you can see from the chart overleaf, is at its highest during the latter part of the first half of the cycle. Oestrogen is responsible for the production of fertile cervical mucus, the opening of the cervix to allow the sperm in to meet the eggs, and the building up of blood in the lining of the uterus, preparing for a fertilized egg.

The cervical mucus is usually very fertile indeed: it is reckoned that sperm can survive for as long as five days in the fertile cervical mucus, waiting for an egg to fertilize. The egg is released from the ovary anything from eight to 14 days from the first day of your cycle – the day your period begins. Ovulation tends to vary from person to person. Some women are aware that they are ovulating as they experience some short-lived pain or stinging sensations in the area of the right or left ovary.

The cells or follicle that protected the egg before it was released remain

THE NORMAL MENSTRUAL CYCLE

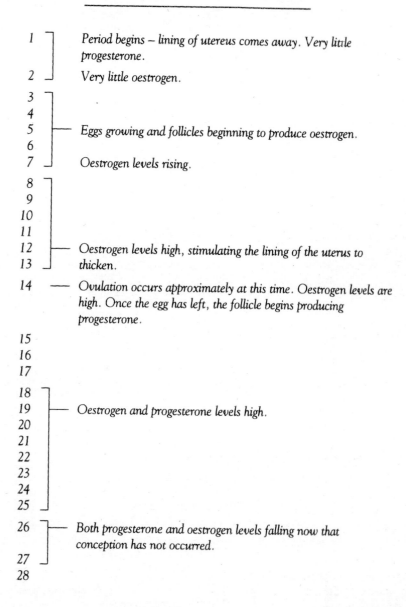

1   *Period begins – lining of utereus comes away. Very little progesterone.*

2   *Very little oestrogen.*

3
4
5   *Eggs growing and follicles beginning to produce oestrogen.*
6
7   *Oestrogen levels rising.*

8
9
10
11
12   *Oestrogen levels high, stimulating the lining of the uterus to*
13   *thicken.*

14   *Ovulation occurs approximately at this time. Oestrogen levels are high. Once the egg has left, the follicle begins producing progesterone.*

15
16
17

18
19   *Oestrogen and progesterone levels high.*
20
21
22
23
24
25

26   *Both progesterone and oestrogen levels falling now that conception has not occurred.*
27
28

in the ovary after the egg has left. The follicle develops into a special gland known as the corpus luteum. Whereas the cells of the follicle were producing large amounts of oestrogen during the first half of the cycle, after ovulation they begin to produce the other important sex hormone, progesterone.

Progesterone is an important hormone at the beginning of pregnancy as it is responsible for producing infertile mucus, preventing sperm and other substances from harming a pregnancy. It is sometimes known as the pregnancy protecting hormone. It also closes the cervix and holds the lining of the uterus in place from ovulation until the next period begins, if fertilization has not taken place. Progesterone levels are sometimes low in women who suffer with PMS, and it has been demonstrated that balancing a woman's nutritional condition can raise the levels of progesterone again. This will be discussed later in the section on nutritional supplements on page 120.

After ovulation the body waits to see whether a pregnancy has occurred. Once it realizes that pregnancy has not occurred, the corpus luteum of the ovary stops working, and the levels of both oestrogen and progesterone fall. As progesterone has been holding the lining of the uterus in place, when this hormone level drops the lining of the uterus is then shed and a menstrual period occurs.

THE MAIN FACTS

Oestrogen controls the first half of the cycle until the egg leaves the ovary, and progesterone is in control of the cycle from the day the egg is released until the menstrual period begins.

The hormones produced by the ovaries have a profound effect on moods and behaviour – not surprising, since oestrogen is a stimulant of the nervous system. Low oestrogen levels cause depression, whereas high oestrogen levels can result in symptoms such as anxiety, irritability and nervous tension. The correct amount of oestrogen produces assertiveness, motivation and emotional stability. Progesterone, on the other hand, is a depressant, and has a calming effect. It is therefore obvious that for a woman to function normally throughout the menstrual cycle a proper balance of these hormones must be maintained.

I will be talking more about how the levels of oestrogen and progesterone are affected by a deficient nutritional state in Chapter 14 on vitamins and minerals, and our laboratory findings. Although it was previously thought that a woman had to take supplements of hormones in

HOW YOUR HORMONAL SYSTEM WORKS

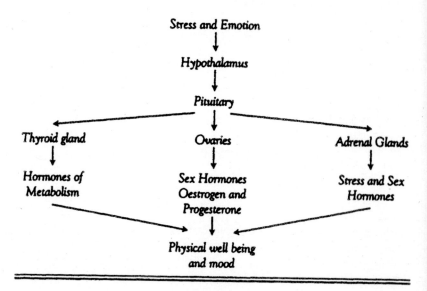

order to maintain her levels if she was deficient, it appears that this is not always so, as you will see.

EFFECTS OF NUTRITION
ON THE MENSTRUAL CYCLE

Nutrition affects the menstrual cycle in many ways. First, there are certain nutrients such as amino acids and vitamins that are necessary for the manufacture of brain hormones and the normal function of the pituitary gland, and which are also capable of influencing moods and behaviour.

Hormones are produced by the ovaries, adrenal glands and the thyroid gland. As already noted, the ovaries produce the sex hormones, oestrogen and progesterone. The adrenal glands produce both sex hormones and hormones related to stress. The thyroid gland produces its own hormones that control the body's rate of metabolism. These three glands – the ovaries, adrenals and thyroid – are all in turn controlled by a part of the brain, the pituitary which, if you like, is the conductor of the hormonal orchestra. It in turn is sensitive to a part of the brain called the hypothalamus which also influences appetite, temperature control and the 24-hour 'biological clock' that controls our eating and sleeping rhythms. It also contains another 'clock' that controls the 28-day menstrual cycle. Finally, it in turn is influenced by levels of stress and emotion. Thus it is that external stress and emotional factors can influence hormonal factors, and ultimately, one's physical sense of well-being and mood.

When an imbalanced diet exists or there are nutritional deficiencies the whole system may become disturbed or more sensitive. If there is a severe reduction in calorie (kj) intake and the body weight falls to an unhealthy level, the function of the pituitary gland will decrease and periods may cease altogether, or may continue but without ovulation. This is nature's way of protecting a woman from becoming pregnant when in an unhealthy state – a rather drastic form of contraception!

The hormones from the pituitary gland, thyroid gland, ovaries and adrenal gland all appear to be influenced slightly by the type of diet you eat, the balance of certain nutrients, exercise and stress. Vitamin B6, vitamin C, zinc, magnesium and other nutrients are subtly involved in the way in which the body responds to or processes the hormones that relate to the normal menstrual cycle. Making sure there is an adequate supply of these essential nutrients from the diet or from the use of supplements is one way to help combat PMS.

Finally, physical and emotional stress can have a powerful effect upon the menstrual cycle. For example, excessive or severe physical exercise, if continued on a regular basis, may cause the pituitary to 'switch off' the ovaries. Thus periods cease and the levels of the sex hormone oestrogen may fall. Such women put themselves at risk of fractures and thinning of the bones – osteoporosis. Emotional stress, such as the worry of becoming pregnant from having unprotected sexual intercourse, can itself lead to the delay or the missing of a period, which in turn causes increased worry and stress – not an uncommon experience at some time in one's life.

So a healthy diet and the avoidance of physical and mental stresses play an important part in health, and especially in the control of Pre-Menstrual Syndrome.

3

PMS DEFINED

PMS, or Pre-Menstrual Syndrome, is the term used to describe a collection of physical and mental symptoms that occur before a period starts and cease with or shortly after the arrival of a period.

WHEN DO SYMPTOMS BEGIN AND END?

- Most commonly symptoms begin from a week to a few days before menstruation begins, and then diminish as the period begins.

- Sometimes symptoms occur at the time of ovulation (mid-cycle), then disappear until a few days pre-menstrually, when they recur until the onset of the period.

- Symptoms may begin at the time of ovulation, around the middle of the cycle, gradually increasing in severity until the period begins. It is not uncommon for symptoms to persist to the first day or two of the period.

WHAT IS THE DIFFERENCE BETWEEN PRE-MENSTRUAL SYNDROME AND PRE-MENSTRUAL TENSION?

- Pre-Menstrual Tension was the original name given to the collection of symptoms relating to tension and anxiety first reported by Dr Frank in the 1930s. Thus the condition became known as 'PMT'.

- Further research was done, particularly by Dr Dalton, who went on to discover further types of symptoms. She renamed the condition Pre-Menstrual Syndrome (PMS).

THE MOST COMMON PMS SYMPTOMS

Have a look at these symptoms. You might be surprised to realize that they are all associated with Pre-Menstrual Syndrome.

Nervous tension	Agoraphobia	Hayfever	Thoughts of
Mood swings	Bad breath	Fatigue	suicide
Irritability	Sensitivity to	Confusion	Sensitivity to
Anxiety	light	Forgetfulness	noise
Depression	Disorientation	Crying	Excessive thirst
Headache	Restlessness	Dizziness	Hostility
Migraine	Mouth ulcers	Tremors and	Sugar cravings
Insomnia	Acne	shakes	
Swollen breasts	Backache	Fainting	Weight gain
Tender/sore	Heart poundings	Asthma	
breasts			
Swollen abdomen	Cramp pains	Loss of interest	Diarrhoea
Bloated feelings	Wind	in sex	Cystitis
Craving for food	Generalized aches	Constipation	
Swelling of	Increased physical	Clumsiness	Boils
extremities	activity	Eczema	Hives
Heavy aching legs	Restless legs	Painful joints	Swollen ankles

JUST KNOWING THAT IT IS PMS

We are often told by patients that just knowing they have an identifiable, not to mention treatable, condition brings much relief in itself. It was a real surprise to me initially to discover women in all walks of life, with varying educational backgrounds, who were under the impression that their symptoms were in one of the following categories:

- All part of being a woman.

- Part of the ageing process.

- Early senile dementia.

- A psychological problem.

- A character fault.

- Schizophrenia.

The chances are that you may have been under an illusion that you fit in to one of these categories. I have lost count of the numbers of women who describe themselves as 'Jekyll and Hyde', i.e. two quite separate people during their menstrual cycle. They all seem to be acutely aware of the change as it occurs some time after ovulation. To a woman, they feel quite powerless to overcome the symptoms.

THE DIFFERENCE BETWEEN
PMS AND PERIOD PAINS

Period pains and other period problems are sometimes wrongly referred to as Pre-Menstrual Syndrome. They are in fact quite different as you will see from the following chart. Despite their differences, we often find that period pains and heavy irregular periods are regulated within four months of following the WNAS programme.

Characteristic	PMS	Period pains
1. Time of onset	3–14 days before period	One day before and/or on first day or two of period
2. Improvement	Approximately the onset of the period	Some time during or at the end of the period
3. After childbirth	Symptoms worsen	Symptoms improve

4

THE MAKING OF PMS

There are a number of factors that may cause or contribute to PMS symptoms. It is very important to examine these thoroughly in order to get the situation into perspective.

GYNAECOLOGICAL OR HORMONAL PROBLEMS

If you have been experiencing problems for some time it is important to consult your doctor for a full check-up. Certainly if you have symptoms that are persistent all month through, there may be other complications present. Here is a small checklist for you to look at to see whether there need be cause for any concern:

Heavy or irregular periods

Abdominal pain

Excessive weight gain or weight loss

Facial hair growth

Persistent severe headaches

Current vaginal discharge, soreness or irritation

Breast lumps or tenderness throughout the menstrual cycle

Milky discharge from the nipples.

If any of these are a current problem it would be advisable to get them checked out, for peace of mind if nothing else. You will then establish whether you have other medical problems as well as PMS, or pure PMS.

FACTORS IN THE CAUSATION OF PMS

1. Difficulty with relationships

2. Problems with work

3. Problem children to cope with

4. Disturbed night's sleep

5. Financial difficulties causing friction and worries

6. Strained relations with husband or partner

7. Inadequate or incorrect diet

8. Eating disorder

9. Environmental pollutants

10. Social poisons

11. Oral contraceptive pill

12. Increasing age, especially age 30–40

13. After childbirth

14. Lack of exercise

15. Operations and physical illnesses

16. After long episodes of breastfeeding

EXAMINING PMS SYMPTOMS

WHAT ACTUALLY CAUSES PMS

In Chapter 2, 'Functioning Normally', hormonal changes throughout the menstrual cycle were described. Whilst major disturbance of hormone levels is not the sole explanation for PMS, certain variations in hormone levels or sensitivity to hormones may well be part of the cause. This in turn can be influenced by stress, dietary factors and nutritional state.

If you are confused about the cause of PMS, don't worry, as most medical scientists and researchers are just as perplexed. Dr Guy Abraham, former Professor of Obstetrics and Gynaecology at the University of California in Los Angeles, has attempted to unravel the causation of PMS by dividing the symptoms into four groups, as detailed below. This somewhat artificial classification does help us to develop possible explanations as to the cause of different aspects of PMS symptoms. Disturbances in the levels of oestrogen and progesterone have been described in some sufferers with different types of PMS, but these are not universal changes. Furthermore, many women will experience symptoms from more than one sub-group.

PMS A (ANXIETY)

This is the most common sub-group. Symptoms are recorded in about 80 per cent of sufferers. The symptoms in this group are:

Nervous tension
Mood swings
Irritability
Anxiety

PMS H (HYDRATION)

This is the second sub-group. It is estimated that symptoms occur in 60 per cent of sufferers. The symptoms in the sub-group are as follows:

Weight gain
Swelling of extremities
Breast tenderness
Abdominal bloating

PMS C (CRAVING)

This is the third sub-group. Symptoms probably occur in 40 per cent of sufferers. There are six symptoms in this sub-group:

Headache
Craving for sweets
Increased appetite
Heart pounding
Fatigue
Dizziness or fainting

PMS D (DEPRESSION)

Of all four sub-groups, this is the one least commonly found on its own. Perhaps 20 per cent of sufferers have PMS D. There are five symptoms in this category:

Depression
Forgetfulness
Crying
Confusion
Insomnia

OTHER SYMPTOMS

Additionally, from our experience with PMS sufferers 13 years ago we identified a further list of common symptoms:

Loss of sexual interest
Disorientation
Clumsiness
Tremors/shakes
Thoughts of suicide
Agoraphobia
Increased physical activity
Heaving/aching legs
Generalized aches
Bad breath
Sensitivity to music/light
Excessive thirst

Each group seems to have different factors involved, except that inadequate diet and stress can be common to all of them. Although some women only suffer with one sub-group of symptoms, it is just as common to be suffering from any combination of sub-groups at the same time. Many severe sufferers seem to have symptoms in all five sub-groups initially.

In the next five chapters I will examine in greater detail each one of these sub-groups of symptoms and look at how the symptoms affected the lives of some of the women who contacted the Women's Nutritional Advisory Service. Rather than describing how PMS might affect various aspects of your life, I decided that the subject might become more alive if it was talked about by sufferers themselves. I have selected patients whose symptoms span a broad spectrum of the Pre-Menstrual Syndrome. By looking into their lives you may well recognize familiar situations.

5

ANXIOUS, IRRITABLE AND UPTIGHT

PMS A (ANXIETY)

The main symptoms of PMS A are nervous tension, anxiety, irritability and mood swings, beginning as early as two weeks before the period and becoming progressively worse as the period approaches.

There are several possible factors, both hormonal and dietary, that might cause pre-menstrual anxiety. Some doctors think that an excess of the hormone oestrogen or an increased sensitivity to it may trigger changes in brain chemistry, resulting in anxiety. The average diet, high in fat and relatively low in fibre, can increase the levels of this hormone. Also, high levels of oestrogen slow down the rate at which the stimulant caffeine is broken down by the liver. This is why some women become more sensitive to tea and coffee when they are pregnant or when taking the oral contraceptive pill.

A lack of vitamin B and possibly the mineral magnesium can also cause changes in the chemistry of the nervous system that can aggravate feelings of anxiety and irritability. Interestingly it seems that some women (and men) who are prone to anxiety and panic attacks are more sensitive to caffeine and genuinely have a more sensitive body metabolism which makes them very susceptible to the effects of a lack of vitamin B or magnesium.

A comparison of caffeine consumption in Chinese nurses and workers in a tea factory revealed a strong association between increased caffeine consumption and the severity of pre-menstrual symptoms. We conducted our own survey in the United Kingdom with *Fitness* magazine which was published in 1992. Three hundred and seventy-seven women took part.

Caffeine consumption was nearly two and a half times higher in PMS sufferers compared with non-sufferers.

On average a mug of tea contains 100 to 130 mg and a mug of coffee between 150 and 250 mg of caffeine. In excess of 250 mg of caffeine can produce symptoms of anxiety, irritability, headache, increased passage of urine and a shaking feeling. Insomnia and palpitations can also occur. It is therefore advisable that these ever popular beverages are limited to just one or two cups or mugs per day and that caffeine-free alternatives are used. More details about these can be found on pages 107–108.

A final and important factor is hyperventilation. This mouthful simply means over breathing. Often when one becomes anxious it is natural to increase the rate and depth of respiration. This provides more oxygen to the bloodstream but also removes more of the waste gas carbon dioxide. This lack of carbon dioxide causes a change in body chemistry which can actually aggravate or cause a variety of symptoms, including numbness and tingling of the fingers, hands and around the mouth, muscle cramps, headaches, light-headedness, increased anxiety, physical and mental fatigue and confusion. The solution is to relax, reduce the rate and depth of breathing and if symptoms are severe to breathe in and out of a paper bag for several minutes. Where these symptoms chronically occur, formal advice and breathing exercises may need to be given by a physiotherapist or psychologist.

ABOUT THE SYMPTOMS

The symptoms in PMS A can at least be disturbing, and at worst feel like a tidal wave of personality change. They are amongst the most common symptoms in PMS.

A staggering 97 per cent of women in our survey of 1000 PMS patients, who were suffering moderately to severely, complained that they suffered to some degree with irritability pre-menstrually, 73 per cent of them with severe irritability, 94 per cent reported mood swings, 64 per cent severe, while 90 per cent reported nervous tension, 54 per cent severe, and 91 per cent reported anxiety, 53 per cent severe.

Degree of irritability suffered out of a sample of 1000 women				
Not Affected	Mild	Moderate	Severe	Total Affected
10%	8%	28%	54% -	90%

As you can imagine, the implications of these figures are fairly devastating. No wonder so many women report Jekyll and Hyde syndrome! Let us look more closely at how PMS A affected the lives of some of our patients.

PMS HITS HOME!

Many women were also reporting wild feelings of violence and aggression pre-menstrually. Their nervous tension seemed to reach uncontrollable peaks, at which time they would lash out at children and husbands or boyfriends. To a woman, they reported that this behaviour was uncharacteristic of them, and that it was having disastrous effects on their families.

The chart below shows to what degree violent and aggressive feelings were a problem. We were very concerned indeed by the result of our research.

Just under 80 per cent of the women studied felt violent or aggressive pre-menstrually. This obviously had serious repercussions on their partners, and on their children in particular.

Sample of 1000 women who admitted being violent/aggressive whilst suffering from PMS				
Not Affected	Once	More Than Once	More Than Six Times	Total Affected
29%	6%	23%	42% -	71%

66 Natasha's Story 99

Natasha is a 38-year-old general practitioner who had suffered from PMS for about seven years. Her symptoms were considerably worse after the birth of her second child.

I felt like a witch

'My worst problems were irritability, bad temper, and being pernickety about things that really didn't matter. I was extremely sensitive to noise and fuss, yelling and snapping at everyone. I felt like a witch, finding everyone else in the family a bother. I could put up with the physical symptoms as long as I felt like "me" the rest of the time and not like "the witch". I felt awful about rows and the yelling at my husband and children. My husband would withdraw into himself and I'd get really frustrated. He used to watch TV or listen to classical music so we talked less. I felt he didn't understand why I was angry and frustrated and I thought we were in a rut. I was always finding reasons for my depression and anger. I was regularly frustrated mid-cycle because I fancied sex but I was so unbearable that my husband obviously didn't. I used to feel that my stress was due to the pressures of having children, the "terrible twos" and so on. Now I'm usually more patient and in less of a hurry, and have time to enjoy them and laugh with them at funny or silly things. Previously I would have been cross with them for slowing me down in the mad rush to get everything done.

I remained fairly in control at work, which I've always enjoyed, so I don't feel that suffered. However, I did have very low self esteem which was usually triggered by comparison to my contemporaries who had become consultants and were working full time as GPs. I used to feel I should have done the same and felt inadequate.

My inability to cope was apparent in other things too. Through lack of co-ordination I pranged the car when parking and dented my bumper – nothing serious thank goodness. I was so forgetful I left the car window open all night: it rained. Another time I left the sunroof open all night: it poured. I drove through red traffic lights; and once I packed the children and shopping into the car and left the buggy in Brighton when I drove off. I would lose things, and I was always bruising myself, bumping into things. PMS is insidious and one doesn't recognize it when it creeps into all aspects of your life. I looked all around me to find causes for the things that were wrong: I blamed my husband, my children, stress and so on. When I look back I find it hard to believe that the centre from which all the bad feelings were emanating was myself. When I was unhappy and desperately seeking a cause, all the time the answer was in my diet.

I had suffered with most of the physical symptoms of PMS. My waist and my bust size would increase before my period, and the day before it started I would pass a lot of urine which led me to believe that a great deal of it was fluid retention. My breasts would swell and as a result I would have to change bra size. At one point I went to the gym to run on a running machine and I had to jog with my arms crossed it was so painful. In the end I invested in a "Cross Your Heart Firm Control Bra" which helped a bit, but it seemed a bit ridiculous as I'm only a 34A bust anyway!

I noticed a change within a month

I tried taking vitamin B6 but it was no use. I abstained from caffeine and chocolate which made a huge difference immediately, but the PMS symptoms returned with the birth of my second child. One day I realized I felt awful almost the whole month. I heard about the WNAS on the radio and found the book Beat PMS Through Diet (the former title of this book) in the library. When I contacted them they put me on a diet which excluded caffeine and chocolate, grains and wheat. I was advised to eat more fresh fruit and vegetables, and to introduce an exercise regime into my life. I took Optivite, Efacal, Efamol, Normoglycaemia, magnesium and linseeds. I noticed the effect of my new regime within a month but still felt a bit precarious. I gradually improved month by month and now PMS is a minor irritation and not a major hurdle every month. I now feel quite normal. I have a few days a month when I'm a bit irritable but I find it easy to deal with. My husband tells me if I'm being a pain and I just shut up! A year ago he wouldn't have dared risk it because I would have sulked for days and felt resentful with a big chip on my shoulder.

The witch has gone

I was beginning to feel, when I was in the midst of PMS, that I was inherently and constitutionally not a very nice person any more. My father used to shout and have a bad temper and I had a secret fear that I was beginning to develop like him as I grew older. The programme has literally given me back my old self: the "witch" has gone. My relationships with my husband and children have improved dramatically. They laugh and joke and tease me a lot now and it is fun! I enjoy my children and don't find them so irritating. Also my mother is now living with us in a relatively small house and we get on really well. We have recenlty moved to quite a remote area, after four years of planning, and my husband and I drove both our cars up

NATASHA

SYMPTOMS

Symptom	WEEK AFTER PERIOD (Fill in 3 days after period)				WEEK BEFORE PERIOD (Fill in 2-3 days before period)			
	None	Mild	Moderate	Severe	None	Mild	Moderate	Severe
PMS - A								
Nervous Tension		✓						✓
Mood Swings		✓					✓	✓
Irritability		✓						✓
Anxiety							✓	
PMS - H								
*Weight Gain	✓					✓		
Swelling of Extremities	✓				✓			
Breast Tenderness	✓					✓		
Abdominal Bloating	✓				✓			
PMS - C								
Headache		✓						✓
Craving for Sweets	✓						✓	
Increased Appetite	✓							✓
Heart Pounding	✓				✓			
Fatigue	✓						✓	
Dizziness or Fainting	✓				✓			
PMS - D								
Depression		✓					✓	
Forgetfulness		✓					✓	
Crying	✓				✓			
Confusion	✓						✓	
Insomnia	✓					✓		
OTHER SYMPTOMS								
Loss of Sexual Interest	✓						✓	
Disorientation	✓				✓			
Clumsiness	✓					✓		
Tremors/Shakes	✓					✓		
Thoughts of Suicide	✓				✓			
Agoraphobia	✓				✓			
Increased Physical Activity	✓					✓		
Heavy/Aching Legs	✓				✓			
Generalized Aches	✓				✓			
Bad Breath	✓				✓			
Sensitivity to Music/Light	✓				✓			
Excessive Thirst	✓				✓			

Do you have any other PRE-MENSTRUAL SYMPTOMS not listed above?

1. Argue with husband then contemplate leaving him and breaking

2. up the marriage – how we'd do it, finances etc.

3. Sensitivity to noise. Find childrens questions and demands

4. unbearably intrusive.

*5. How much weight do you gain before your period? _____

FOLLOW UP
PRE-MENSTRUAL SYNDROME QUESTIONNAIRE

Name: Natasha   Age: 37   Height: 5' 2"   Weight: 9st 5lb

MARITAL STATUS: Single _____   Married ✓   Divorced _____   Widowed _____

(Please tick where applicable)

PRESENT CONTRACEPTION: None _____   Pill _____   I.U.D _____   Other ✓

Your periods come every __27-28__ days   Your periods last _____ days

Your periods are: Light _____   Moderate _____   Heavy _____

SYMPTOMS	WEEK AFTER PERIOD (Fill in 3 days after period)				WEEK BEFORE PERIOD (Fill in 2-3 days before period)			
	None	Mild	Moderate	Severe	None	Mild	Moderate	Severe
PMS - A								
Nervous Tension	✓					✓		
Mood Swings	✓				✓			
Irritability	✓					✓		
Anxiety	✓				✓			
PMS - H								
*Weight Gain	✓				✓			
Swelling of Extremities	✓				✓			
Breast Tenderness	✓					✓		
Abdominal Bloating	✓				✓			
PMS - C								
Headache	✓				✓			
Craving for Sweets	✓				✓			
Increased Appetite	✓					✓		
Heart Pounding	✓				✓			
Fatigue	✓				✓			
Dizziness or Fainting	✓				✓			
PMS - D								
Depression	✓				✓			
Forgetfulness	✓				✓			
Crying	✓				✓			
Confusion	✓				✓			
Insomnia	✓				✓			
OTHER SYMPTOMS								
Loss of Sexual Interest	✓				✓			
Disorientation	✓				✓			
Clumsiness	✓				✓			
Tremors/Shakes	✓				✓			
Thoughts of Suicide	✓				✓			
Agoraphobia	✓				✓			
Increased Physical Activity	✓				✓			
Heavy/Aching Legs	✓				✓			
Generalized Aches	✓				✓			
Bad Breath	✓				✓			
Sensitivity to Music/Light	✓				✓			
Excessive Thirst	✓				✓			

on a two-day journey with the children, my mother, two cats that had never met before – and I coped! We have had to make new friends and I have started a new job. All round, we have been through a lot of changes, and we've managed together. We've laughed together at things that have gone wrong. When the PMS had been at its worst, I couldn't have coped, my husband couldn't possibly have put up with me, and everyone would have suffered. Thank you WNAS.'

Natasha's follow-up questionnaire after four months on page 25 looks dramatically different. She had a few mild symptoms remaining which may have been partly due to the fact that the sale of her house fell through and life was a bit stressful.

From a letter Natasha sent at the end of her programme you can see that her husband feels he has got back the girl he married which speaks for itself. Life has once again become enjoyable.

It's been 16 years since I started the WNAS programme. Comparing now with then, the biggest change is that now I feel content with life and often I'm happy and really enjoying things. Then I woke up every morning with a feeling of dread, wondering how I was going to get through the day, awful tiredness, and I found everything was getting to be rather a struggle. My patience was minimal and everything was an irritation. The slightest thing would trigger off what felt like an instant personality change and I'd be in "witch" mode: unpleasant, cutting, sarcastic – it makes me shiver to remember it. In this state I smacked my elder daughter far too hard on several occasions.

My husband said that in my worst tempers I used to go on about breaking up, and he would go out of the room without saying anything and hope I'd shut up or calm down. I remember my mind coldly running along those lines and working out how we'd split the house and the children and so on. My husband simply says that at last he's got back the woman that he married.

I've changed my diet considerably and I now avoid all grains except rice and barley and I try to eat much more fruit and vegetables. I don't eat chocolate any more and I don't drink tea or coffee. I really miss toast, hot-cross buns, pizza and chocolate but I'd much rather be my normal happy easygoing self, so I'm not tempted. I also take Optivite, Efamol and Normoglycaemia, magnesium and linseeds.

Many thanks for sorting me out and helping to put PMS where it belongs – as a minor monthly irritation – instead of a problem that was dominating my life by affecting my thinking and altering my character and all my relationships.

Natasha Burton

" Sarah's Story "

Sarah was another member of the medical profession who had been suffering with PMS since she was a teenager. She was a 37-year-old nurse with two young children who felt normal for only one week in her cycle: three quarters of her life was disrupted by her PMS.

'Having PMS was like being held under water in the dark, panicking and trying to breathe. I would desperately try to work out why my life was in such a mess. But no matter what I did, nothing seemed to help. Then, as if by magic and at the click of a finger, my period arrived and I was up out of the water and into the light. I became my old self again, happy, confident, optimistic, loving me and everyone; this would last for at least a week. Then all too soon I began to be slowly pushed back down, to tread water for another three weeks and go through the same ordeal all over again.

I suffered from the usual symptoms of PMS: terrible bloating; swollen breasts when my bra would feel incredibly tight; headaches; heavy sweats; and bad breath around period time. But the worst symptoms of all were the constant anxiety and palpitations. I would sweat heavily, especially when in any social situation such as school trips, shopping or with chance callers. I was unable to remember the word for an object or a person's name, and they might even be a member of my family! I had this weird feeling of being me and trying to stop myself feeling so horrid, but just not being able to stop. I would suffer terrible depressions, and the most awful violent, verbal rages which would leave me with a sore throat.

I have nearly crashed the car several times in the midst of me doing my screaming raving looney bit at my children. A week prior to my period I would notice an increase in the need for sweet foods, always around four o'clock. I would often buy a bar of chocolate before picking up the children from school. Once home I would just stuff anything I could get hold of: three to four slices of toast with jam, masses of bsicuits, all with coffee, and still have a meal with dessert.

My husband was very supportive, and on and off I would enjoy our sex life together and was pleased I had made the effort, but if my husband had a heavy work load, I would be happy just to let it go. I was always unpredictable, I could wake up and be nice, and end up screaming at the children because the house was in a mess. I would just excuse it by saying to everyone that I couldn't cope. This makes for a very tense family.

People at work irritated me beyond reason and I would be incredibly snappy. If I was involved with a project, I would be hyperactive in short

SARAH

SYMPTOMS

	WEEK AFTER PERIOD (Fill in 3 days after period)				WEEK BEFORE PERIOD (Fill in 2-3 days before period)			
	None	Mild	Moderate	Severe	None	Mild	Moderate	Severe
PMS - A								
Nervous Tension	✓							✓
Mood Swings	✓							✓
Irritability	✓							✓
Anxiety	✓							✓
PMS - H								
*Weight Gain	✓					✓		
Swelling of Extremities	✓					✓		
Breast Tenderness	✓						✓	
Abdominal Bloating	✓						✓	
PMS - C								
Headache	✓					✓		
Craving for Sweets	✓					✓		
Increased Appetite						✓		
Heart Pounding	✓						✓	
Fatigue	✓						✓	
Dizziness or Fainting	✓					✓		
PMS - D								
Depression	✓				✓			
Forgetfulness	✓							✓
Crying							✓	
Confusion	✓							✓
Insomnia	✓						✓	
OTHER SYMPTOMS								
Loss of Sexual Interest	✓					✓		
Disorientation	✓				✓			
Clumsiness	✓					✓		
Tremors/Shakes	✓					✓		
Thoughts of Suicide	✓				✓			
Agoraphobia	✓				✓			
Increased Physical Activity	✓						✓	
Heavy/Aching Legs	✓						✓	
Generalized Aches	✓					✓		
Bad Breath	✓				✓			
Sensitivity to Music/Light	✓							✓
Excessive Thirst	✓						✓	

Do you have any other PRE-MENSTRUAL SYMPTOMS not listed above?

1. <u>I sweat in unfamiliar social situations</u>

2. <u>I have tendency to stammer</u>

3. <u>Irrational behaviour</u>

4. _____

*5. How much weight do you gain before your period? <u>2-3 lbs</u>

bursts. Everything was all or nothing and I would be totally exhausted. I'd be quite together, though, as far as my work was concerned, keeping my irritation to myself as much as I could until I got home, where I screamed and ranted at my family.

I hated myself

My doctor prescribed progesterone tablets and pessaries, and I'd be OK for a while but then my breasts would swell, I'd have swollen ankles and breakthrough bleeding. I was on these for over seven months and then he suggested that I go on a mixture of oestrogen and testosterone. I felt a total failure and I hated myself. I hated being the one causing the upset around our home and I felt everything was my fault.

Then a friend gave me a copy of the book, Beat PMS Through Diet (the former title of this book) and I contacted the WNAS, hardly believing that someone knew and understood my symptoms and how to treat them. They put me on a special diet: no gluten, cutting out cafeine, and eating lots more fruit and vegetables. I was also asked to exercise at least three times a week. I was to take supplements of Optivite, Efamol and Normoglycaemia every day.

In one month I felt much better, but I didn't know how much better I could feel until another month had passed. And now I feel just brilliant! It's like being given a new lease of life; I feel like a new woman. I know this sounds very sad, but in the early days, the contrast to the raving looney I used to be made me cry with the sheer joy and amazement of what simple things like food, vitamins and diet can do for a girl.

Life is wonderful

I was bogged down in the mess of my PMS, and it got to the stage where I dreaded the onset of my symptoms. I was sick to death of myself, sick of worrying, moaning and crying. I was sick of this raving looney of a woman I had become. After being given Maryon Stewart's book I have never looked back. I now take exercise which I thoroughly enjoy. I'm finding out about my body and how exhilarating it can be to own one! I'm so laid back with my children they think it's Christmas every day. I make time for a social life and I don't see everything as a big deal, so I arrange things in advance and not at the last minute. I always have a meal cooked every day which is a great leap forward for me and an absolute treat for the family. I have even started a new career – I'm retraining to be a chiropodist. I can now read books and concentrate and actually follow the story line, which I couldn't before. I have much more patience, and I pamper myself more. In short, I'm having a wonderful life!'

FOLLOW UP
PRE-MENSTRUAL SYNDROME QUESTIONNAIRE

Name: Sarah _____ Age: _____ Height: _____ Weight: _____

MARITAL STATUS: Single _____ Married _____ Divorced _____ Widowed _____

(Please tick where applicable)

PRESENT CONTRACEPTION: None _____ Pill _____ I.U.D _____ Other _____

    Your periods come every _____ days   Your periods last _____ days

    Your periods are: Light _____ Moderate _____ Heavy _____

SYMPTOMS

	WEEK AFTER PERIOD (Fill in 3 days after period)				WEEK BEFORE PERIOD (Fill in 2-3 days before period)			
	None	Mild	Moderate	Severe	None	Mild	Moderate	Severe
PMS - A								
Nervous Tension	✓				✓			
Mood Swings	✓				✓			
Irritability	✓				✓			
Anxiety	✓				✓			
PMS - H								
*Weight Gain	✓					✓		
Swelling of Extremities	✓					✓		
Breast Tenderness	✓				✓			
Abdominal Bloating	✓				✓	✓		
PMS - C								
Headache	✓				✓			
Craving for Sweets	✓				✓			
Increased Appetite	✓				✓			
Heart Pounding	✓				✓			
Fatigue	✓				✓			
Dizziness or Fainting	✓				✓			
PMS - D								
Depression	✓				✓			
Forgetfulness	✓				✓			
Crying	✓				✓			
Confusion	✓				✓			
Insomnia	✓				✓			
OTHER SYMPTOMS								
Loss of Sexual Interest	✓				✓			
Disorientation	✓				✓			
Clumsiness	✓				✓			
Tremors/Shakes	✓				✓			
Thoughts of Suicide	✓				✓			
Agoraphobia	✓				✓			
Increased Physical Activity	✓				✓			
Heavy/Aching Legs	✓				✓			
Generalized Aches	✓				✓			
Bad Breath	✓				✓			
Sensitivity to Music/Light	✓				✓			
Excessive Thirst	✓				✓			

Sarah struggled with her symptoms for most of her menstruating life. She describes herself as a 'raving loony' and admits that her behaviour obviously affected her relationship with her husband and her family life. Classically, when her period began all her symptoms went.

She had tried a wide selection of medical treatments to help ease her symptoms and every self-help approach she was able to lay her hands on but her symptoms still persisted.

Her follow-up questionnaire (page 30) reflects the degree of progress she made. Most of her symptoms have completely gone – just a bit of mild weight gain and bloating remains on the day before her period.

End result

'Since undertaking the nutritional programme to overcome my PMS, I can honestly say my symptoms have disappeared. I think they have really vanished, like absolute magic. I am overwhelmed by it. My life is now back to normal. There is no comparison in me now. I am a completely different woman. Back to what I was before.'

Sarah's letter to me at the end of her programme describes how desperate she was to find a cure for her PMS. Knowing her now as an exxtremely vivacious character it seems hard to believe that just a short time ago she felt that life held so little for her.

Dear Maryon,

I believe that looking back over my past history of raving loony moments, they have always been under the influence of pre-menstrual tension. Even I was, for many years, under the impression that it could be ignored, and it would go away. How wrong I was, and what misery it caused.

When my raving loony moments began to dominate my life and that of all those around me, I knew I had to do something, because I would shout and scream at the children and rant and rave until I couldn't speak. I would cry a lot. I couldn't remember things, appointments, the name of objects, what I went upstairs for, how to get from A to B. I couldn't face people, and when I had to see and talk to them I would sweat and stammer and often get palpitations. I put on weight, so I felt like Mrs Blobby. All this does nothing for a girl's self esteem.

I used to have three weeks of feeling like this and only one week of being normal. I tried all the usual media panacea and supposedly miracle cures – vitamin B6, Evening Primrose Oil, exercise until it nearly killed me – then seven months of hormone treatment. This gave me enormous breasts, which was frankly foolish and unnecessary, as I had an ample supply.

So I was on the hunt again, but determined to find a solution. I was moaning to a fellow sufferer who gave me your book, and as they say, "I have never looked back". Here at last was the answer, and it worked. My PMS type was identified and I got on with my new diet, exercise and supplement plan. I came off wheat, barley, oats, rye. Off tea, coffee, coke and chocolate. And on to corn, Rooi-bosh tea, green salads, oily fish, bio-yoghurt, loads of fruit. Four lots of exxercise per week. Finally Optivite tablets (multi-vitamin), Evening Primrose Oil (Efamol) and Normoglycaemia tablets (helps control sugar levels).

So I believe I've done really well for an ex-raving loony. I'm now the person I always was, the one that was in prison for three weeks out of each month. Having turned the tables I have my life back, and I'm having a wonderful life, thanks to Maryon, Alan and everyone at the WNAS.

66 Maureen's Story 99

Maureen is a 47-year-old nursing lecturer in further education whose moods were so wildly out of control that she was in the process of disciplinary action at work and finding life generally difficult.

'I had experienced symptoms for nearly 25 years, but they had become markedly worse in the last three years. My doctor had prescribed numerous forms of hormone treatment which seemed to make the symptoms worse. My irritability, anger and aggression had almost totally alienated me from the world. I was struggling along, continuously taking the contraceptive pill as my doctor felt my symptoms would improve if we could suppress ovulation.

Suicide seemed attractive

I had a great deal of time off in the last three years because of my wild moods. Things got so bad at work I even had to see the occupational health doctor as the personnel department needed his reassurance that I could cope with my job. I had been off work for three months in two consecutive years due to my symptoms so there was a general feeling that I was on my way out. At the time, I was struggling to look after 30 students and I could never imagine having my own team.

I had reached the point where I was afraid to go out of the house. I was so tired that I could not get out of bed in the morning without a friend phoning *to command me through the procedure limb by limb. My doctor had sent me for counselling and had even referred me to a psychiatrist, but I walked out halfway through the appointment as I was so angry with him. I often felt like ending my life. I had upset so many people and had lost most of my friends. At work I was treated with caution and regarded as an oddity.*

I read about this book in Woman and Home magazine and decided to read it. To my utter amazement my mood changes were described almost exactly by other case histories. I made some changes to my diet myself by following the instructions in the book while I was waiting for my appointment with the WNAS. There I was asked to make considerable changes to my diet. I cut out certain grains, caffeine and biscuits, which I used to eat day and night. I also took supplements of Optivite and went back to exercising, which I had let slip from my routine.

At my follow-up appointment, six weeks later, I was able to report that I had been on an even keel with no wild mood swings. I could hardly believe it and nor could my friends and colleagues. I came off the pill, too, and my headaches and utter fatigue also disappeared.

Within three months I had lost half a stone (3 kg) in weight; I was wonderfully stable each day and had regained my enthusiasm for life. I had renewed my friendships, applied to do an MA in education which had been a goal I never dared hope for, and within one month was promoted to co-ordinator at work. It has now been two years since my treatment with the WNAS and I even manage to cope well with my stressful job. These days I am responsible for 150 students. I won the hospital contract to train qualified staff nurses to be NVQ assessors. I am actively involved in training and research and have managed to develop a successful research package which is now being implemented in our local area. Considering that not so many years ago I was lurching from one day to the next not knowing what the future holds, I am extremely happy with the outcome. I went to see my doctor last month following a car accident. It was the first time I had seen him in two years whereas in the old days he was monitoring me weekly because he was deeply concerned. My sense of humour has returned and I have renewed my friendships. I feel alive again and can't sing the praises of the WNAS enough.'

Maureen is a single woman who has not had any children. Nevertheless, at the time she came to us she had been suffering with PMS symptoms for some 25 years. Maureen's fear was that she would lose her job and, in fact, almost did. She had had so many months off because of her symptoms that she was hardly able to perform her duties at work as you saw on page 32. She is now a very creative leader of a large team implementing new methods that she has pioneered into her work, which is something that

MAUREEN

SYMPTOMS

	WEEK AFTER PERIOD (Fill in 3 days after period)				WEEK BEFORE PERIOD (Fill in 2-3 days before period)			
	None	Mild	Moderate	Severe	None	Mild	Moderate	Severe
PMS - A								
Nervous Tension	✓							✓
Mood Swings	✓						✓	
Irritability	✓						✓	✓✓
Anxiety		✓					✓	
PMS - H								
*Weight Gain		✓						✓
Swelling of Extremities	✓							
Breast Tenderness	✓							
Abdominal Bloating		✓						✓
PMS - C								
Headache	✓							✓
Craving for Sweets	✓						✓	
Increased Appetite	✓						✓	
Heart Pounding	✓					✓		
Fatigue			✓					✓
Dizziness or Fainting	✓					✓		
PMS - D								
Depression		✓					✓	
Forgetfulness	✓					✓		
Crying	✓							✓
Confusion	✓						✓	
Insomnia	✓						✓	
OTHER SYMPTOMS								
Loss of Sexual Interest	✓							
Disorientation								
Clumsiness	✓							
Tremors/Shakes	✓						✓	
Thoughts of Suicide	✓						✓	
Agoraphobia	✓							
Increased Physical Activity	✓							
Heavy/Aching Legs	✓						✓	
Generalized Aches	✓							
Bad Breath	✓							
Sensitivity to Music/Light	✓						✓	
Excessive Thirst	✓					✓		

Do you have any other PRE-MENSTRUAL SYMPTOMS not listed above?

1. _____

2. _____

3. _____

4. _____

*5.   How much weight do you gain before your period?   3-4 lbs

FOLLOW UP
PRE-MENSTRUAL SYNDROME QUESTIONNAIRE

Name: Maureen   Age: 48   Height: _____   Weight: _____

MARITAL STATUS: Single _____   Married _____   Divorced _____   Widowed _____

(Please tick where applicable)

PRESENT CONTRACEPTION: None _____   Pill _____   I.U.D _____   Other _____

    Your periods come every _____ days   Your periods last _____ days

    Your periods are: Light _____   Moderate _____   Heavy ✓

SYMPTOMS	WEEK AFTER PERIOD (Fill in 3 days after period)				WEEK BEFORE PERIOD (Fill in 2-3 days before period)			
	None	Mild	Moderate	Severe	None	Mild	Moderate	Severe
PMS - A								
Nervous Tension	✓				✓			
Mood Swings	✓				✓			
Irritability	✓				✓			
Anxiety	✓				✓			
PMS - H								
*Weight Gain	✓				✓			
Swelling of Extremities	✓				✓			
Breast Tenderness	✓				✓			
Abdominal Bloating	✓				✓			
PMS - C								
Headache	✓				✓			
Craving for Sweets	✓					✓		
Increased Appetite	✓				✓			
Heart Pounding	✓				✓			
Fatigue	✓				✓			
Dizziness or Fainting	✓				✓			
PMS - D								
Depression	✓				✓			
Forgetfulness	✓				✓			
Crying	✓				✓			
Confusion	✓				✓			
Insomnia	✓				✓			
OTHER SYMPTOMS								
Loss of Sexual Interest	✓				✓			
Disorientation	✓				✓			
Clumsiness	✓				✓			
Tremors/Shakes	✓					✓		
Thoughts of Suicide	✓				✓			
Agoraphobia	✓				✓			
Increased Physical Activity	✓				✓			
Heavy/Aching Legs	✓				✓			
Generalized Aches	✓				✓			
Bad Breath	✓				✓			
Sensitivity to Music/Light	✓				✓			
Excessive Thirst	✓				✓			

she never dared dream of. You will see that there is a dramatic difference between her before and after charts on pages 34 and 35 and two years later she remains well and happy. Problem areas were the tension and anxiety symptoms, and the swelling and bloating symptoms, as you can see from her chart overleaf.

Understandably, she was frightened about the effect that her ever-recurring symptoms had on her body and on her life. All areas of her life were disrupted because of her symptoms, and despite trying a series of treatments, both independently, and through her doctor, her symptoms showed no sign of easing off. The thought of going through her whole life suffering in this manner had been pretty uncomfortable to Maureen.

6

BLOATING, WEIGHT GAIN AND BREAST TENDERNESS

PMS H (HYDRATION)

PMS H sufferers complain of weight gain pre-menstrually. The hands and feet often swell so that rings and shoes become too tight. The face often becomes puffy and the waistline expands so that clothes feel too tight. The abdomen can become bloated and tender and the same applies to the breasts.

The manifestations of these symptoms are mostly physical, in that women report feeling very uncomfortable and often sore. Because of their increased size many women feel self-conscious and get very touchy and introverted. Surprisingly, most women who suffer from PMS H only gain up to 3–4 pounds (1–2 kg) pre-menstrually. Approximately 20 per cent seem to gain far more than this. I have personally seen women who gain up to 12 pounds (5.4 kg) before their periods. They literally change dress size and need to have two sets of underwear to cope with their increased breast size.

Symptoms due to excess fluid retention can easily be worsened by eating the wrong diet. A high intake of sodium or ordinary salt, which is the norm in the United Kingdom, is the commonest cause of fluid retention in women. It appears that some women are particularly prone to develop fluid retention whereas others can eat salty foods with impunity. Thus part of the programme for those with fluid retention symptoms is to greatly reduce the intake of salt from that used in the cooking, that added to food at the table and from salty foods. Nowadays, like our consumption of sugar, at least two-thirds of the salt we eat is 'hidden' in common foods such as bacon, ham, sausages, other preserved meat products, cheeses, most butters and margarines, bread, tinned foods like tinned tuna and vegetables, salted crisps and nuts and most savoury snacks and convenience meals.

Good old plain fruit and vegetables, meat, fish, beans and rice are all low in sodium and have good levels of potassium. A good intake of potassium and magnesium from the diet may help minimize the effects of too much sodium. Fortunately there are many low-salt (sodium) versions of tinned and other foods now available.

Consuming a lot of carbohydrate-rich foods and sugar, including that from soft drinks, which many women drink in substantial quantities pre-menstrually, can also lead to fluid retention. Curiously, drinking a lot of water, low-calorie drinks and even tea and coffee without sugar does not cause this problem. Losing weight if you are overweight may also help with fluid retention symptoms.

However, some women who complain of pre-menstrual abdominal bloating and puffy fingers do not have an increase in body water and salt content. It may be that their perception of their body changes and they just 'feel' different.

THE DEGREE OF SUFFERING

In our survey we found that 90.8 per cent of the women complained of abdominal bloating to some degree (72 per cent severe to moderately).

Of the women studied 86.8 per cent had pre-menstrual breast tenderness (67 per cent severe to moderate sufferers).

Weight was gained by 84 per cent (52 per cent severe to moderately) and 54 per cent complained of swelling of the extremities (33 per cent severe to moderate).

**Degree of pre-menstrual
breast tenderness
suffered out of a sample
of 1000 women**

Not Affected	Mild	Moderate	Severe		Total Affected
18%	24%	26%	32%	-	82%

Degree to which abdominal bloating affected a sample of 1000 women pre-menstrually					

Not Affected	Mild	Moderate	Total Severe		Affected
12%	15%	37%	36%	-	88%

WEIGHT LOSS

Whilst conducting our follow-up consultations during the programme and in our clinics, we began to notice that many overweight women who were previously unable to lose weight were enthusiastically reporting weight loss. This began occurring even after the first month, without even 'dieting' to lose weight. In fact, their intake of food during the programme was in many cases greater than usual.

Because of this somewhat unexpected outcome, we decided to monitor a group of 50 PMS sufferers who were also overweight, through the first three months of their programme. (Thirty-six of the women were at least 10 per cent overweight and 14 of them were obese, which means greater than 33 per cent above normal body weight.) The symptoms complained of most severely to begin with were weight gain, fatigue, abdominal bloating, craving for food, in particular sweet foods, and anxiety.

After three months on their programmes there was an 84 per cent reduction in severe symptoms.

The overweight group of 36 women lost an average of 7 pounds (3 kg) and the obese group of 14 women lost an average of 13 pounds (6 kg) in this three-month period.

We can't say precisely why this amount of weight loss had occurred, particularly when the women had previously found it difficult to lose weight. However, the common denominator seems to be that they were all on a healthy diet that had been balanced according to their individual needs. We therefore suspect that this must have had a positive effect on their metabolism with the result that they began to shed excess weight.

This is certainly an area we would like to research further. But in the meantime it's a gift horse that won't be looked in the mouth by PMS H sufferers.

" Julie's Story "

Julie is a 33-year-old PE teacher from Sussex who suffered with aggression and anger as well as migraine and other PMS symptoms for 17 years. She was diagnosed as having IBS in 1991. Her symptoms were so severe that her job was on the line, and her relationship with her husband and her social life were also in jeopardy.

Violent feelings that knew no bounds

'I suffered with PMS for years and IBS was diagnosed two years before I met up with the WNAS in 1993. I had been married for five years to a very supportive husband, but my behaviour and mood swings got really extreme. I was very irrational, smashing things and was very violent towards my 15 stone (95 kg) husband which really frightened me. I really felt I could kill, and my language was so blue which was incredibly uncharacteristic. I was on the pill for ten years during which my periods were lighter, but in the ten or so days leading up to my periods I would get awful migraines. Once I was sick and fainted at school, and I even crashed the car pre-menstrually.

An irritable bowel

As well as this, the Irritable Bowel Syndrome I suffered was severe and embarrassing. I had loud tuning noises in my stomach, diarrhoea and even had awful accidents when I was out; it was like being incontinent and I would just pass froth. I was obsessed with the fear that it would happen when I was taking a lesson and I would have to run off and leave the children. It became even worse around period time. Despite being given the medical "all clear", I was convinced that I had bowel cancer. I went off sex and I was in such a state; my poor husband really suffered. I wanted to have a child but I was too frightened to even try to conceive while I was in this condition. In truth, I thought I would never be free of my symptoms, which was both frightening and depressing.

My mother read about the WNAS in Good Housekeeping magazine. She passed the article to my husband who read it and strongly advised me to go for treatment. He wanted some peace! He wanted his friend back.

At my appointment I was given a programme to follow which involved cutting out orange juice, tea, cola and chocolate, and eating more fruit and vegetable fibre and oily fish. In addition I took a multi-vitamin and mineral supplement, and while I had always done a lot of exercise in my job as a PE

JULIE

SYMPTOMS	WEEK AFTER PERIOD (Fill in 3 days after period)				WEEK BEFORE PERIOD (Fill in 2-3 days before period)			
	None	Mild	Moderate	Severe	None	Mild	Moderate	Severe
PMS - A								
Nervous Tension			✓					✓
Mood Swings			✓					✓
Irritability		✓						✓
Anxiety		✓					✓	
PMS - H								
*Weight Gain	✓					✓		
Swelling of Extremities	✓					✓		
Breast Tenderness		✓				✓		
Abdominal Bloating	✓					✓		
PMS - C								
Headache	✓						✓	
Craving for Sweets		✓						✓
Increased Appetite	✓						✓	
Heart Pounding	✓				✓			
Fatigue		✓					✓	
Dizziness or Fainting	✓					✓		
PMS - D								
Depression		✓						✓
Forgetfulness	✓					✓		
Crying	✓							✓
Confusion	✓						✓	
Insomnia	✓				✓			
OTHER SYMPTOMS								
Loss of Sexual Interest		✓						✓
Disorientation	✓				✓			
Clumsiness	✓					✓		
Tremors/Shakes	✓				✓			
Thoughts of Suicide	✓						✓	
Agoraphobia	✓				✓			
Increased Physical Activity		✓			✓			
Heavy/Aching Legs	✓				✓			
Generalized Aches	✓					✓		
Bad Breath	✓				✓			
Sensitivity to Music/Light	✓					✓		
Excessive Thirst	✓					✓		

Do you have any other PRE-MENSTRUAL SYMPTOMS not listed above?

1. Incredible strength – e.g. can pick up my 15-stone husbamd

2. Violent towards my husband; loss of judgement while in a rage.

3. Scream and shout. Feel the cold more. Feel unwanted and

4. unloved. Irritable bowel syndrome worsens.

*5. How much weight do you gain before your period?   1-2 lbs

41

PRE-MENSTRUAL SYNDROME QUESTIONNAIRE

Name: Julie   Age: 30   Height: 5' 9"   Weight: 11st 4lb

MARITAL STATUS: Single _____   Married ✓   Divorced _____   Widowed _____
(Please tick where applicable)

PRESENT CONTRACEPTION: None ✓   Pill _____   I.U.D _____   Other _____

    Your periods come every __erratic__ days   Your periods last __2-3__ days

    Your periods are: Light ✓   Moderate _____   Heavy _____

SYMPTOMS

	WEEK AFTER PERIOD (Fill in 3 days after period)				WEEK BEFORE PERIOD (Fill in 2-3 days before period)			
	None	Mild	Moderate	Severe	None	Mild	Moderate	Severe
PMS - A								
Nervous Tension	✓					✓		
Mood Swings	✓					✓		
Irritability	✓					✓		
Anxiety	✓				✓			
PMS - H								
*Weight Gain	✓					✓		
Swelling of Extremities	✓				✓			
Breast Tenderness	✓				✓			
Abdominal Bloating	✓				✓			
PMS - C								
Headache	✓					✓		
Craving for Sweets	✓					✓		
Increased Appetite	✓				✓			
Heart Pounding	✓				✓			
Fatigue	✓				✓			
Dizziness or Fainting	✓				✓			
PMS - D								
Depression	✓				✓			
Forgetfulness	✓				✓			
Crying	✓				✓			
Confusion	✓				✓			
Insomnia	✓				✓			
OTHER SYMPTOMS								
Loss of Sexual Interest	✓				✓			
Disorientation	✓				✓			
Clumsiness	✓				✓			
Tremors/Shakes	✓				✓			
Thoughts of Suicide	✓				✓			
Agoraphobia	✓				✓			
Increased Physical Activity	✓					✓		
Heavy/Aching Legs	✓				✓			
Generalized Aches	✓				✓			
Bad Breath	✓				✓			
Sensitivity to Music/Light	✓				✓			
Excessive Thirst	✓					✓		

teacher I tried to increase my personal exercise and relaxation regime.

Within two months my symptoms were under control and within six months I was feeling wonderful. No diarrhoea, no IBS at all and even the PMS had gone. My husband is thrilled. He has been so helpful when you think of what he's been through. I am amazed that these symptoms are overcome naturally. I'm not feeling murderous anymore my energy level has increased, and to cap it all when I lose my temper – no swearing!

In 1993 I had our first baby, Mary-Kate, and am in very good health. My hormones are stable and I had a very good pregnancy and amazingly easy birth. For the first six months I was very relaxed about what I ate but now I'm back on the diet and taking my supplements. I'm back to my fighting weight and feeling really on top of things. No matter what some doctors say, it does matter what you put into your body. It is so obvious that it is frequently overlooked. I haven't looked back, and now I value my happy family situation even more, knowing only too well what might have been.'

Apart from the mental symptoms that Julie experienced pre-menstrually, which made her feel extremely anti-social, she also had to suffer the embarrassment of her PMT H symptoms. Every day was a nightmare as she was afraid that she would embarrass herself and not make it to the toilet in time. She lived in hope that there would be a solution to her problem but was not confident that she would ever experience relief before undertaking the WNAS programme. Her follow-up questionnaire on page 42 really speaks for itself. Several years after following the programme she remains well and is able to live life to the full.

❝ Claire's Story ❞

After 11 years of suffering for three weeks out of four with totally unpredictable mood swings and utterly debilitating physical symptoms, plus extreme cravings for chocolate pre-menstrually which are mentioned further on page 56, Claire has managed to get herself back to being a normal wife, lover and mother. Claire had also been extremely accident prone as you will see on page 92. Despite the fact she has a disabled child she is able to remain cheerful and supportive to others around her.

Dear Maryon,

I am writing to thank you for all your help and guidance in treating my PMS. Life has improved greatly since I started the programme. By taking supplements, regular exercise and watching my diet I remain well.

The family have all noticed a great improvement in my behaviour towards them and are much more relaxed around me. I am no longer aggressive and nasty towards them. In the mornings when I wake I now see the sunshine and not the dark, ugly cloud that bought misery into all our lives.

Life at present is busy and stresseful at times. Philip has now found work but the hours are long and it's not unusual for him to be working 16 hours in one shift. So life is pretty full with one thing and another, but on the positive side I would never have been able to cope if I had not addressed my PMS symptoms. I am really indebted to you.

Yours sincerely,
Claire

CLAIRE

SYMPTOMS	WEEK AFTER PERIOD (Fill in 3 days after period)				WEEK BEFORE PERIOD (Fill in 2-3 days before period)			
	None	Mild	Moderate	Severe	None	Mild	Moderate	Severe
PMS - A								
Nervous Tension		✓						✓
Mood Swings	✓							✓
Irritability		✓						✓
Anxiety	✓						✓	
PMS - H								
*Weight Gain	✓						✓	
Swelling of Extremities	✓						✓	
Breast Tenderness	✓						✓	
Abdominal Bloating	✓						✓	
PMS - C								
Headache	✓				✓			
Craving for Sweets	✓							✓
Increased Appetite	✓							✓
Heart Pounding	✓				✓			
Fatigue	✓						✓	
Dizziness or Fainting	✓					✓		
PMS - D								
Depression	✓							✓
Forgetfulness		✓						✓
Crying	✓					✓		
Confusion	✓						✓	
Insomnia	✓				✓			
OTHER SYMPTOMS								
Loss of Sexual Interest	✓				✓			
Disorientation	✓					✓		
Clumsiness	✓					✓		
Tremors/Shakes	✓					✓		
Thoughts of Suicide	✓						✓	
Agoraphobia	✓							✓
Increased Physical Activity	✓						✓	
Heavy/Aching Legs	✓							✓
Generalized Aches	✓						✓	
Bad Breath	✓				✓			
Sensitivity to Music/Light			✓					✓
Excessive Thirst	✓							✓

Do you have any other PRE-MENSTRUAL SYMPTOMS not listed above?

1.   Sensitivity to noise

2.

3.

4.

*5.   How much weight do you gain before your period?   5 lbs approx

45

FOLLOW UP
PRE-MENSTRUAL SYNDROME QUESTIONNAIRE

Name: Claire   Age: 35   Height: 5' 4"   Weight: 10st 8lb

MARITAL STATUS: Single ✓   Married ✓   Divorced _____   Widowed _____

(Please tick where applicable)

PRESENT CONTRACEPTION: None _____   Pill _____   I.U.D _____   Other sheath

    Your periods come every __28__ days   Your periods last __5-7__ days

    Your periods are: Light _____   Moderate _____   Heavy ✓

SYMPTOMS

	WEEK AFTER PERIOD (Fill in 3 days after period)				WEEK BEFORE PERIOD (Fill in 2-3 days before period)			
	None	Mild	Moderate	Severe	None	Mild	Moderate	Severe
PMS - A								
Nervous Tension	✓							
Mood Swings	✓				✓			
Irritability	✓				✓			
Anxiety	✓				✓			
PMS - H								
*Weight Gain	✓				✓			
Swelling of Extremities	✓				✓			
Breast Tenderness	✓				✓			
Abdominal Bloating	✓				✓			
PMS - C								
Headache	✓				✓			
Craving for Sweets	✓					✓		
Increased Appetite	✓					✓		
Heart Pounding	✓				✓			
Fatigue	✓				✓			
Dizziness or Fainting	✓				✓			
PMS - D								
Depression	✓				✓			
Forgetfulness	✓				✓			
Crying	✓				✓			
Confusion	✓				✓			
Insomnia	✓				✓			
OTHER SYMPTOMS								
Loss of Sexual Interest	✓				✓			
Disorientation	✓				✓			
Clumsiness	✓				✓			
Tremors/Shakes	✓				✓			
Thoughts of Suicide	✓				✓			
Agoraphobia	✓				✓			
Increased Physical Activity	✓				✓			
Heavy/Aching Legs	✓				✓			
Generalized Aches	✓				✓			
Bad Breath	✓				✓			
Sensitivity to Music/Light	✓				✓			
Excessive Thirst	✓				✓			

7

SUGAR CRAVINGS, HEADACHES AND FATIGUE

PMS C (CARBOHYDRATE CRAVING)

In this sub-group of PMS, one to two weeks before the period the appetite increases. Cravings for food begin, particularly for sweet foods and chocolate. Often stress intensifies the situation. Satisfying the cravings is a vicious circle. A typical example is as follows.

The day starts with either no breakfast or just a couple of cups of tea or coffee and a few cigarettes. This may stimulate the body's metabolism and one's energy for a short while, but the problems begin by mid-morning. By this time the energy level tends to fall, and symptoms of nervousness, anxiety, palpitations, light headaches, hunger and cravings for food, particularly sweet foods, set in. Another cup of tea or coffee with sugar, or with a sugary or chocolate snack, may delay symptoms for a while but nothing short of a good wholesome meal will resolve these symptoms.

Some of these symptoms may be due to a fall in the level of sugar (glucose) in the blood – known as hypoglycaemia. As the brain and nervous system rely upon glucose for their source of energy, a fall in its level can cause a whole host of nervous system symptoms. The body compensates by producing adrenaline, which increases the level of glucose in the blood, but aggravates symptoms of anxiety, palpitations, sweating and shaking.

Such symptoms may be improved by the next meal. Often the mid-morning or mid-afternoon fatigue or sweet cravings are relieved by a wholesome lunch, supper or snack. What is not widely appreciated is that our calorie requirements in our premenstrual week increase by up to 500 calories per day – which is a staggering amount. The body has a genuine need for more wholesome food at this time and failure to provide it results in savings in blood sugar levels.

Not all women will have such marked symptoms, nor indeed will there always be marked swings in blood sugar levels. Often one just feels better if one eats three good meals a day, a couple of healthy snacks, and has a regular, not too hectic lifestyle.

Headaches can also be caused by excessive intake of tea and coffee. Fatigue can be affected by the balance of minerals, such as iron and magnesium. Any woman with persistent fatigue should certainly see her doctor for examination and appropriate blood tests, particularly to check for anaemia or reduced activity of the thyroid gland.

GOOD FOOD REGULARLY, PLEASE!

So often the cravings for sweet foods, sugary snacks and chocolate are the result of an irregular and inadequate diet. Women with PMS C – carbohydrate cravings – may also experience headache, increased appetite, heart pounding, fatigue, and dizziness and fainting. These symptoms can be due to the swings in blood sugar levels and over-reliance on social stimulants: caffeine from tea, coffee, cola, chocolate, alcohol, cigarettes and even marijuana. Three good, regular meals, two wholesome in-between-meal snacks and cutting down on sugar and social stimulants are all essential to treat PMS C.

THE DEGREE OF SUFFERING

In our study we found that 77 per cent of the women were suffering with cravings for sweet food, just over 60 per cent severe to moderately. There were 93 per cent who reported suffering with fatigue pre-menstrually, 82 per cent severe to moderately; 77 per cent reported headaches premenstrually, 74 per cent general increased appetite, 53 per cent heart pounding and 50 per cent dizziness and fainting.

" Cheryl's Story "

Cheryl is a 35-year-old mother of three and a company secretary who has suffered from PMS since the birth of her third child in 1989.

'I was put on the pill at 15 to control my periods. I used to have days off work each month as my periods were so painful. After I had my third baby my husband was sterilized and I didn't need to take the pill any more. But my PMS symptoms got worse and worse. For half of my cycle I would have mood swings and be really irritable. My husband would retreat and batten down the hatches in an attempt to avoid confrontation. About a week before my period I would have terrible breast tenderness and bloating, which was so bad it looked as though I was pregnant.

I felt like a chocolate pig

I suffered from headaches, back and stomach cramps and went mad for anything sweet like chocolate. I could quite happily eat five or six bars of chocolate a day sometimes, and then go looking for more. I ate a whole packet of seven Penguins and do you know, I didn't even taste them. I'd go out from work at lunchtime in my pre-menstrual week and eat at least five bars of chocolate in the hour, while everyone else was still on their first.

They hid from me

All my family were experts at disappearing at certain times of the month when it was obvious that Mum was on a short fuse. Whenever I lost my temper, screaming and shouting, either they would vanish or I would lock myself in the bathroom and have a good cry. My husband had a timetable when he could safely broach things and when he couldn't! He was really good, very supportive really but our sex life suffered because sometimes I honestly couldn't be bothered. I just felt so low, asking myself why no one understood what was happening to me. It was a real nightmare; we had 14 days of living normally and 14 days of hell.

Then by pure chance I caught Maryon Stewart of the WNAS on GMTV and bought the book Beat PMS Through Diet (the former title of this book) straight away. I approached the WNAS and was put on their programme: a diet with no wheat, caffeine, chocolate, sugar or salt. It was quite a challenge as I am a vegetarian but I was given detailed advice about what to eat and drink. Plus I took nutritional supplements and started an exercise programme.

CHERYL

SYMPTOMS	WEEK AFTER PERIOD (Fill in 3 days after period)				WEEK BEFORE PERIOD (Fill in 2-3 days before period)			
	None	Mild	Moderate	Severe	None	Mild	Moderate	Severe
PMS - A								
Nervous Tension	✓						✓	
Mood Swings	✓							✓
Irritability	✓							✓
Anxiety	✓							✓
PMS - H								
*Weight Gain	✓						✓	
Swelling of Extremities	✓				✓			
Breast Tenderness	✓							✓
Abdominal Bloating	✓						✓	
PMS - C								
Headache	✓							✓
Craving for Sweets	✓						✓	
Increased Appetite	✓						✓	
Heart Pounding	✓						✓	
Fatigue	✓							✓
Dizziness or Fainting	✓						✓	
PMS - D								
Depression	✓							✓
Forgetfulness	✓				✓			
Crying	✓							
Confusion	✓				✓			
Insomnia	✓				✓			
OTHER SYMPTOMS								
Loss of Sexual Interest	✓							✓
Disorientation	✓				✓			
Clumsiness	✓				✓			
Tremors/Shakes	✓				✓			
Thoughts of Suicide	✓					✓		
Agoraphobia	✓				✓			
Increased Physical Activity	✓				✓			
Heavy/Aching Legs	✓				✓			
Generalized Aches	✓					✓		
Bad Breath	✓				✓			
Sensitivity to Music/Light	✓				✓			
Excessive Thirst	✓						✓	

Do you have any other PRE-MENSTRUAL SYMPTOMS not listed above?

1. backache

2. _____

3. _____

4. _____

*5. How much weight do you gain before your period? 2-4 lbs

FOLLOW UP
PRE-MENSTRUAL SYNDROME QUESTIONNAIRE

Name: Cheryl   Age: 35   Height: 5' 7"   Weight: 10st 12lb

MARITAL STATUS: Single _____   Married ✓   Divorced _____   Widowed _____

(Please tick where applicable)

PRESENT CONTRACEPTION: None ✓   Pill _____   I.U.D _____   Other _____

    Your periods come every __28__ days   Your periods last __5-7__ days

    Your periods are: Light ✓   Moderate ✓   Heavy _____

SYMPTOMS	WEEK AFTER PERIOD (Fill in 3 days after period)				WEEK BEFORE PERIOD (Fill in 2-3 days before period)			
	None	Mild	Moderate	Severe	None	Mild	Moderate	Severe
PMS - A								
Nervous Tension	✓				✓			
Mood Swings	✓				✓			
Irritability	✓				✓			
Anxiety	✓				✓			
PMS - H								
*Weight Gain	✓					✓		
Swelling of Extremities	✓				✓			
Breast Tenderness	✓				✓			
Abdominal Bloating	✓					✓		
PMS - C								
Headache	✓				✓			
Craving for Sweets	✓				✓			
Increased Appetite	✓				✓			
Heart Pounding	✓				✓			
Fatigue	✓				✓			
Dizziness or Fainting	✓				✓			
PMS - D								
Depression	✓				✓			
Forgetfulness	✓				✓			
Crying	✓				✓			
Confusion	✓				✓			
Insomnia	✓				✓			
OTHER SYMPTOMS								
Loss of Sexual Interest	✓				✓			
Disorientation	✓				✓			
Clumsiness	✓				✓			
Tremors/Shakes	✓				✓			
Thoughts of Suicide	✓				✓			
Agoraphobia	✓				✓			
Increased Physical Activity	✓				✓			
Heavy/Aching Legs	✓				✓			
Generalized Aches	✓				✓			
Bad Breath	✓				✓			
Sensitivity to Music/Light	✓				✓			
Excessive Thirst	✓				✓			

Life is now a doddle

I began my programme in December 1996 and after two months I was surprisingly well. When I had my third period I just sailed through it with no symptoms. It was a doddle! I'd say I was 110 per cent better. I have no period problems now or any PMS symptoms. Our sex life has improved dramatically. My husband is enjoying the experience of this new woman! He was away on a diving holiday and he came back expecting the worst as usual, but I was amazed to find that I'd coped extremely well in his absence and everything was fine, we were all in one piece. I have no more cravings, no temper tantrums. I do an hour's exercise daily so even the dog benefits. I was a demon on legs before my period and now I'm so calm it's not true. I'm feeling brilliant!'

One of Cheryl's particular weaknesses was her craving for sweet food premenstrually and her excessive indulgence. Later on in Chapter 11, I will be talking about the detrimental effects of excessive amounts of sweet food, particularly in relation to PMS symptoms.

On her first chart Cheryl's worst symptoms were in the sub-groups PMS A and PMS C, although she did have symptoms in all four categories.

Interestingly, Cheryl didn't even like the taste of chocolate despite the fact that she was eating so much and sometimes ate it so quickly she couldn't even taste it.

Like the majority of women, Cheryl was lacking in education about the importance of a correct diet. This is hardly surprising considering how little we learned at school about nutrition as a subject. Until recent times very little attention has been placed on the role of nutrition in relation to women's health.

'I knew a bit about diet, but had no idea that changing my diet could bring me back to normal, and that's what it has done. Although I didn't know that I was sensitive to any foods, I had a good idea what was and what wasn't a sensible diet. My trouble was temptation. It's much easier to buy chocolate, which is available wherever you go, than it is to go home and make fish cakes with sesame seeds on them or things like that which you know are much better for you. I did eat healthy things, but I also ate a load of rubbish.

I try to stick to the diet. I feel much better when I do. I know I shouldn't eat chocolates, processed food, salty food or wheat. I did try some Stilton cheese and crisps, but I blew up like a balloon shortly after eating them. I now know that chocolate makes me depressed and, of course, I put on weight if I eat rubbish.

End result

Since I've been following the nutritional programme I feel so much better. My children notice the difference in me; I am no longer nasty to them. It has made me feel so much better in myself. I personally feel fine, although I could still do with losing weight.

I still have my marital problems. But I know that we have got things wrong marriage-wise, I know they are not related to PMS. I haven't got that aggressiveness inside me so much and I haven't got that awful feeling, that black cloud hanging over my head. That was the worst thing.'

Cheryl's follow-up charts show that she overcame her symptoms completely and as an added bonus she got back her libido which had been gone for some time and was placing a strain on her relationship. You can read more about this on page 72.

Another victim of chocolate cravings was Gail Brown who was a 36-year-old working mother of two young children. She had been suffering with uncontrollable pre-menstrual bingeing since she finished breastfeeding her younger child. She also started to suffer from very heavy periods as well as PMS.

❝ Gail's Story ❞

'I've always been a vegetarian; very health conscious and sporty. Not the type you'd think would suffer from PMS. But that all changed after I had my second baby. When my periods returned it was with a vengeance. I never understood why menstruation was called "the curse" by some women but then I had been lucky enough to have periods as regular as clockwork which were completely trouble free.

After my son was born in 1989 my periods gradually became problematic. Over the following 18 months they became so bad that for the first two days of each period I felt as if I was having a haemorrhage. I tried to be light-hearted but it was hard not to be frightened and upset by the colossal loss of blood. The blood loss remained heavy and clotted for the entire duration of my period and as a result I hardly left the house; I started to feel imprisoned by my hormones.

I needed a fix

During this time I had also developed pretty unpleasant symptoms before my

GAIL

SYMPTOMS	WEEK AFTER PERIOD (Fill in 3 days after period)				WEEK BEFORE PERIOD (Fill in 2-3 days before period)			
	None	Mild	Moderate	Severe	None	Mild	Moderate	Severe
PMS - A								
Nervous Tension		✓					✓	
Mood Swings	✓							✓
Irritability		✓						✓
Anxiety	✓					✓		
PMS - H								
*Weight Gain		✓						✓
Swelling of Extremities	✓					✓		
Breast Tenderness	✓				✓			
Abdominal Bloating		✓					✓	
PMS - C								
Headache	✓				✓			
Craving for Sweets		✓						✓
Increased Appetite		✓						✓
Heart Pounding	✓				✓			
Fatigue		✓						✓
Dizziness or Fainting	✓				✓			
PMS - D								
Depression	✓						✓	
Forgetfulness		✓					✓	
Crying	✓					✓		
Confusion	✓					✓		
Insomnia	✓				✓			
OTHER SYMPTOMS								
Loss of Sexual Interest	✓							✓
Disorientation	✓				✓			
Clumsiness	✓				✓			
Tremors/Shakes	✓					✓		
Thoughts of Suicide	✓				✓			
Agoraphobia	✓				✓			
Increased Physical Activity			✓		✓			
Heavy/Aching Legs	✓				✓			
Generalized Aches	✓				✓			
Bad Breath	✓				✓			
Sensitivity to Music/Light	✓					✓		
Excessive Thirst	✓				✓			

Do you have any other PRE-MENSTRUAL SYMPTOMS not listed above?

1. Bruising appears above and below eyes/swelling and dryness over

2. bridge of nose.

3. _____

4. _____

*5. How much weight do you gain before your period? 4-7 lbs

FOLLOW UP
PRE-MENSTRUAL SYNDROME QUESTIONNAIRE

Name: Gail _____ Age: 36 ____ Height: 5' 3½" ___ Weight: 9st 8lb ____

MARITAL STATUS: Single ____ Married ✓ Divorced _____ Widowed _____

(Please tick where applicable)

PRESENT CONTRACEPTION: None ✓ Pill ____ I.U.D ____ Other ____

Your periods come every __26-28__ days   Your periods last __5-6__ days

Your periods are: Light _____ Moderate _____ Heavy ✓

SYMPTOMS	WEEK AFTER PERIOD (Fill in 3 days after period)				WEEK BEFORE PERIOD (Fill in 2-3 days before period)			
	None	Mild	Moderate	Severe	None	Mild	Moderate	Severe
PMS - A								
Nervous Tension	✓				✓			
Mood Swings	✓				✓			
Irritability	✓					✓		
Anxiety	✓				✓			
PMS - H								
*Weight Gain	✓				✓			
Swelling of Extremities	✓				✓			
Breast Tenderness	✓				✓			
Abdominal Bloating	✓				✓			
PMS - C								
Headache	✓				✓			
Craving for Sweets	✓				✓			
Increased Appetite	✓				✓			
Heart Pounding	✓				✓			
Fatigue	✓				✓			
Dizziness or Fainting	✓				✓			
PMS - D								
Depression	✓				✓			
Forgetfulness	✓				✓			
Crying	✓				✓			
Confusion	✓				✓			
Insomnia	✓				✓			
OTHER SYMPTOMS								
Loss of Sexual Interest	✓				✓			
Disorientation	✓				✓			
Clumsiness	✓				✓			
Tremors/Shakes	✓				✓			
Thoughts of Suicide	✓				✓			
Agoraphobia	✓				✓			
Increased Physical Activity	✓				✓			
Heavy/Aching Legs	✓				✓			
Generalized Aches	✓				✓			
Bad Breath	✓				✓			
Sensitivity to Music/Light	✓				✓			
Excessive Thirst	✓				✓			

period. The irritability and mood swings became progressively worse and worse. On one memorable occasion I remember banging my head against the wall to stop myself from hitting my own child. Throughout all this, my husband remained very supportive, but terribly worried and concerned. By this time I felt so ill for two weeks before my period I couldn't even hold down my job as a personal assistant in my husband's firm. It was really frightening and sometimes I felt like I was totally losing control. I also found myself craving bars of chocolate and junk food. At first it was one or two bars of chocolate a week, but within months, I was sometimes eating five or six chocolate bars after the evening meal. My craving for chocolate was insatiable and I was eating only junk food.

Gail was a real 'chocoholic'. Fortunately, we were able to relieve her of these cravings early on in her programme. Over the years we have had great success treating cravings for sweet food. If this is your main problem you may be interested to read about the latest research and how to overcome the problems in the book *Beat Sugar Craving*. See page 274 for details.

" Claire's Story "

You will remember from Claire's story on page 43 that she was battling with her symptoms and life. The fuel on the fire was her chocolate addiction.

I had extreme sugar cravings and it wasn't unusual on a very bad day, to get through three packets of chocolate biscuits each containing 15 to 18 biscuits. Extras included Bounty; Mars bars; bars of chocolate; and lots of coffee, usually with the biscuits. At the worst I was having coffee every half hour. Forty minutes or so after eating the chocolate treats, I would become depressed and so eat more chocolate. It was a vicious circle.

8

DEPRESSION, CRYING AND THOUGHTS OF SUICIDE

PMS D (DEPRESSION)

Depression is a common pre-menstrual symptom and usually is present with other symptoms such as anxiety and breast tenderness. Our own research has shown that those most likely to suffer from pre-menstrual depression are more often overweight and do less exercise than those who do not suffer so badly with this problem.

The balance of certain nutrients has an important influence on both hormone and brain chemistry. Magnesium, for example, influences how the ovaries respond in the normal menstrual cycles, and many other nutrients are also important in this respect. It is also known that in people with severe depression the chance of finding some degree of B vitamin deficiency is much higher than would be expected in the general population. These nutrients have been used successfully in treating both PMS and depression.

In our study we found that 90 per cent of the women suffered from pre-menstrual depression, 75 per cent severe to moderately. This, we felt, was a frighteningly high number, and in view of the possible consequences of depression, not something that should be taken lightly.

Degree to which 1000 women suffered depression pre-menstrually				
Not Affected	Mild	Moderate	Severe	Total Affected
10%	15%	19%	56% -	90%

In 1959 Dr Katharina Dalton published a study in the *British Medical Journal* which showed that the time of admission to hospital of depressed patients coincided with the menstrual period, the pre-menstrual phase, and ovulation.

The balance of hormones – or whatever determines their balance, seems to be crucial in controlling mood. We are beginning to learn how diet and lifestyle can influence our hormones and our moods.

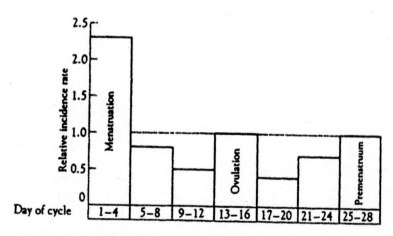

Time of admission of 185 patients with depression.
(*From Dalton K. (1959). Br. Med. J.; 1:148–149.*)

SUICIDAL

Many women who were suffering with PMS D reported that they felt suicidal, indeed it was because we were coming across so many women who felt suicidal that we decided to embark on the study of 1,000 women.

Tragically, we found that 52 per cent of them had previously contemplated suicide pre-menstrually, 39 per cent of them several times and 9 per cent had actually attempted suicide pre-menstrually. A staggering 90 women out of the 1,000 that were chosen.

Suicidal tendencies out of a sample of 1000 women				
Once	More than once	More than six times	Total contemplated	Attempted
13%	25%	14%	52%	9%

A group of French doctors have linked attempted suicide in the pre-menstrual phase with low levels of the hormone oestrogen. However, some of the women had normal or even high levels of this hormone. For some an imbalance in this hormone might affect brain chemistry and thus mood. A healthy diet, exercise, nutritional supplements and controlling stress are the types of approaches that can help normalize hormone and body chemistry and thus decrease pre-menstrual depression.

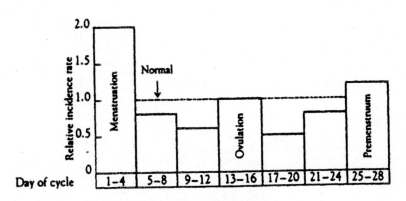

Time of acute psychiatric admission in 276 patients.
(From Dalton K. (1959). Br. Med. J.; 1:148–149.)

Again in 1959 Dr Dalton looked at the timing of 276 acute psychiatric admissions in four London hospitals. According to her findings, which were published in the *British Medical Journal*, 46 per cent of the patients were admitted between the 25th day of their cycle and the 4th day of their new cycle.

Also 53 per cent of attempted suicides, 47 per cent of admissions for depression and 47 per cent of schizophrenic patients were admitted during these eight days of the menstrual cycle.

66 Marilyn's Story 99

Marilyn is a 23-year-old single woman who works as a medical secretary. She suffered with PMS for four years and described her symptoms as a monthly battle. Just before beginning our programme she kept a diary of her symptoms and has given us permission to quote an extract from it. You will see from her diary that Marilyn's PMS symptoms turned her into a zombie each month. We could be forgiven for thinking that such a patient had serious psychological problems rather than straightforward PMS.

Diary of a PMS sufferer

'I am afraid that my fears have been realized again this month, as it has turned out to be one of the worst episodes that I have had for months.

My head feels heavy and I seem to be walking around in a daze. Days are passing with little memory or recollection. At the beginning of the day I wonder how I will make it through, but I somehow manage to. I have lapses between wishing to be on my own, and almost dreading being with others, for fear that my anxieties will overcome perspectives and develop into an unwanted and distressing panic attack. Then at times I need to be with people that I am close to, for I need their support and reassurance and the calming factor which they give to me. I have made a promise to myself that I will not allow my body and my mind to endure this destructive illness which turns a normal person into some kind of monster. The people I love suffer and are tormented with me as a result of my symptoms.'

Marilyn had become so depressed that she was contemplating suicide. She spent half of her life in a tearful daze and the other half bewildered as to why her personality changed so dramatically before her period.

MARILYN

SYMPTOMS	WEEK AFTER PERIOD (Fill in 3 days after period)				WEEK BEFORE PERIOD (Fill in 2-3 days before period)			
	None	Mild	Moderate	Severe	None	Mild	Moderate	Severe
PMS - A								
Nervous Tension		✓						✓
Mood Swings	✓							✓
Irritability	✓							✓
Anxiety		✓						✓
PMS - H								
*Weight Gain	✓				✓			
Swelling of Extremities	✓					✓		
Breast Tenderness	✓					✓		
Abdominal Bloating	✓						✓	
PMS - C								
Headache	✓				✓			
Craving for Sweets	✓							✓
Increased Appetite	✓					✓		
Heart Pounding	✓						✓	
Fatigue	✓							✓
Dizziness or Fainting	✓						✓	
PMS - D								
Depression	✓							✓
Forgetfulness	✓							✓
Crying	✓							✓
Confusion	✓						✓	
Insomnia	✓					✓		
OTHER SYMPTOMS								
Loss of Sexual Interest	✓					✓		
Disorientation	✓						✓	
Clumsiness	✓						✓	
Tremors/Shakes	✓						✓	
Thoughts of Suicide	✓					✓		
Agoraphobia	✓						✓	
Increased Physical Activity	✓					✓		
Heavy/Aching Legs	✓					✓		
Generalized Aches	✓						✓	
Bad Breath	✓					✓		
Sensitivity to Music/Light	✓						✓	
Excessive Thirst	✓					✓		

Do you have any other PRE-MENSTRUAL SYMPTOMS not listed above?

1. I sometimes experience higher than normal temperatures.

2. _____

3. _____

4. _____

*5. How much weight do you gain before your period? _____

FOLLOW UP
PRE-MENSTRUAL SYNDROME QUESTIONNAIRE

Name: Marilyn   Age: 23   Height: 4' 10"   Weight: 6st 8lb

MARITAL STATUS: Single ✓   Married ____   Divorced ____   Widowed ____
(Please tick where applicable)

PRESENT CONTRACEPTION: None ____   Pill ✓   I.U.D ____   Other ____

Your periods come every __24__ days   Your periods last __5__ days

Your periods are: Light ✓   Moderate ____   Heavy ____

SYMPTOMS

	WEEK AFTER PERIOD (Fill in 3 days after period)				WEEK BEFORE PERIOD (Fill in 2-3 days before period)			
	None	Mild	Moderate	Severe	None	Mild	Moderate	Severe
PMS - A								
Nervous Tension	✓				✓			
Mood Swings	✓				✓			
Irritability	✓				✓			
Anxiety	✓				✓			
PMS - H								
*Weight Gain	✓				✓			
Swelling of Extremities	✓				✓			
Breast Tenderness	✓				✓			
Abdominal Bloating	✓				✓			
PMS - C								
Headache	✓				✓			
Craving for Sweets	✓				✓			
Increased Appetite	✓				✓			
Heart Pounding	✓				✓			
Fatigue	✓				✓			
Dizziness or Fainting	✓				✓			
PMS - D								
Depression	✓				✓			
Forgetfulness	✓				✓			
Crying	✓				✓			
Confusion	✓				✓			
Insomnia	✓				✓			
OTHER SYMPTOMS								
Loss of Sexual Interest	✓				✓			
Disorientation	✓				✓			
Clumsiness	✓				✓			
Tremors/Shakes	✓				✓			
Thoughts of Suicide	✓				✓			
Agoraphobia	✓				✓			
Increased Physical Activity	✓				✓			
Heavy/Aching Legs	✓				✓			
Generalized Aches	✓				✓			
Bad Breath	✓				✓			
Sensitivity to Music/Light	✓				✓			
Excessive Thirst	✓				✓			

Life had nothing to offer

'My PMS suffering was slowly getting worse and lasting for more days as the months rolled past. My doctor prescribed the contraceptive pill which I took for three years but it didn't seem to make any difference. I still experienced panic attacks every month, I was extremely anxious, weepy and tearful and wondered what life really had to offer. In the days before my period I would wrongly blame and accuse others, and misconceive what they had to say. Those who are close to me bore the brunt of my accusations as I truly believed that they really didn't love me. People didn't, through various acceptable reasons, fit in with exxactly what I wanted, but then I would accuse them of selfishness when maybe I should have been looking closer to home. When I read about the work of the WNAS in a women's magazine it seemed like a dream come true. I dreamt of not only getting my life back but also my dignity. I used to be considered to be a cheerful person but that seems so long ago. In fact, while my boyfriend went away two years ago I seriously contemplated suicide. Fortunately I came to my senses in time.

I was very impressed with the progress I made after following the WNAS programme for the first month. I even managed to stay off chocolate and be reasonably pleasant to everyone I came into contact with. During my second month I had a couple of set backs, as my car was written off while I was parked and sitting in it, and then I went down with gastro-enteritis. By the following month I was back on track and I really haven't looked back since, except that when I tried to reintroduce chocolate I became very moody and depressed again.

I don't notice my periods at all now. I have no pain, no pre-menstrual symptoms, I feel healthy and not possessed by anyone else, and I feel as if I have truly overcome my monthly battle.'

By comparing Marilyn's before and after charts you will see that her former irrational and depressive behaviour had been replaced by health and well being. She is no longer a slave to her PMS and is able to enjoy her work life and her personal relationships.

PMS D can be very severe indeed. We have dealt with some very sad cases, where women felt suicidal, depressed and that life was not worth living pre-menstrually.

The first example I will give you is the story of Grace Edwards.

❝   Grace's Story   ❞

Grace is a 36-year-old carer who is married with four children. She has been suffering from PMS for 18 years, and it had become worse in the last year. Her doctor had prescribed Prozac and had arranged for her to see a psychiatrist. She was subsequently given hormone treatment and sent to see a second psychiatrist who suggested she took Librium.

I felt so incapable

'For almost the whole month I felt awful. I was withdrawn, depressed and anti-social. I often thought of suicide and I'd lock myself away, not even wanting to see my children. I used to rant and rave at them, and then feel really guilty. It got so bad that my mother-in-law would come to take the children away at the weekends to give me a break. I gave up my job eventually because of my symptoms, and even kept one of the children away from school to look after the baby as I was ridden with panic attacks and felt totally incapable.

Why couldn't I be a normal mother?

My boss was very kind and understanding, but my doctor, when I went to him in tears and told him it might be something to do with my periods, raised his eyes and told me to increase the dose of the Prozac. All the family were feeling the strain, and although my husband was very supportive, even he got to the point where he said "That's enough!" – after I had laid into the children again on one occasion. My relationship with my children was so poor it hurt me a great deal. I'd watch mothers with their children and think "Why can't that be me?"

My new diet

A relative had a copy of the book Beat PMS Through Diet (the former title of this book). I contacted the WNAS and started on the programme at the end of April 1995. I had to make big changes to my diet, cutting out wheat, tea and coffee, and taking supplements. But it really was worth it. I noticed progress in the first month, but I still had bad days. In June, my doctor suggested I take hormones in order to stop my periods altogether and go backon to the anti-depressants to help my palpitations. I didn't take his advice, but carried on with the programme.

By August 1995 my symptoms had disappeared. I cannot believe that I am the same person – I have got my life back. I tore up the prescription for hormones, stopped taking anti-depressants, lost a stone (6 kg) in weight while on the programme and am now working during the day and some evenings, and going to college! My husband thinks it's marvellous. I am a different person. Before, I didn't want to be bothered about anything, but *now I feel brilliant. I spend so much more time with my children and they really love it, particularly the family cycling trips. This is the real me.'*

Grace not only sounded as though she should see a psychiatrist but was in fact sent to see two. The drugs that she was prescribed would, at best, have masked her symptoms had they worked and would certainly not have addressed the root cause. She made a remarkable transformation and is immensely grateful.

PMT D symptoms can be particularly frightening and isolating, especially when it seems that the profession has little more to offer.

It is not just women who have had children who suffer with severe symptoms of PMT D, Janet is a classic example of a career women who held down a demanding job as a senior analyst. She had suffered with severe depression or bouts of irrational anger for over a year, and had suffered with PMS generally before she went on the pill at the age of 17.

❝ Janet's Story ❞

I knew I was wildly out of control

'I had been with my husband for about eight years and we had a really good relationship, but it was very hard for him to cope with my behaviour. My interest in sex had waned too. My problems in general began years before, and had increased to the point where I would suffer for three weeks of my cycle, building up to my period. I would have severe mood swings, anxiety, palpitations, depression and forgetfulness, as well as breast tenderness, craving for sweet things, and feeling dizzy and faint when I didn't eat. I could ignore sweet things generally, but something would happen to throw me and I would reach for the chocolates and biscuits, sometimes eating five bars of chocolate at a time. I had one week out of three when I was free of all these things. I was at an all-time low.

I really felt that if I hadn't had such a crisis at work in January last year, PMS would have wrecked my life. I'd been suffering from chronic depression at the time and had a couple of drinks at work before telling my colleagues, mostly men, to get lost. They packed me into a taxi and I came home convinced that I'd been right to do it. Now I see it as a severely irrational outburst. My workmates knew that it was not like me to be depressed or aggressive and were completely stunned. It was suggested I sign off for a while to get myself sorted out.

JANET

SYMPTOMS

	WEEK AFTER PERIOD (Fill in 3 days after period)				WEEK BEFORE PERIOD (Fill in 2-3 days before period)			
	None	Mild	Moderate	Severe	None	Mild	Moderate	Severe
PMS - A								
Nervous Tension	✓							✓
Mood Swings	✓						✓	
Irritability	✓							✓
Anxiety	✓						✓	
PMS - H								
*Weight Gain	✓						✓	
Swelling of Extremities	✓					✓		
Breast Tenderness	✓							✓
Abdominal Bloating	✓					✓		
PMS - C								
Headache	✓				✓			
Craving for Sweets	✓					✓		
Increased Appetite		✓						✓
Heart Pounding	✓				✓			
Fatigue		✓						✓
Dizziness or Fainting		✓						✓
PMS - D								
Depression	✓							✓
Forgetfulness		✓						✓
Crying	✓						✓	
Confusion	✓					✓		
Insomnia	✓					✓		
OTHER SYMPTOMS								
Loss of Sexual Interest	✓				✓			
Disorientation	✓				✓			
Clumsiness	✓					✓		
Tremors/Shakes	✓						✓	
Thoughts of Suicide	✓				✓			
Agoraphobia	✓				✓			
Increased Physical Activity		✓				✓		
Heavy/Aching Legs	✓							✓
Generalized Aches		✓					✓	
Bad Breath	✓							✓
Sensitivity to Music/Light	✓				✓			
Excessive Thirst		✓						✓

Do you have any other PRE-MENSTRUAL SYMPTOMS not listed above?

1. Sinusitis

2. Aggression

3. Acne

4.

*5. How much weight do you gain before your period? 5 lbs

FOLLOW UP
PRE-MENSTRUAL SYNDROME QUESTIONNAIRE

Name: Janet _____ Age: _____ Height: _____ Weight: _____

MARITAL STATUS: Single _____ Married _____ Divorced _____ Widowed _____

(Please tick where applicable)

PRESENT CONTRACEPTION: None _____ Pill _____ I.U.D _____ Other _____

Your periods come every _____ days   Your periods last _____ days

Your periods are: Light _____   Moderate _____   Heavy _____

SYMPTOMS	WEEK AFTER PERIOD (Fill in 3 days after period)				WEEK BEFORE PERIOD (Fill in 2-3 days before period)			
	None	Mild	Moderate	Severe	None	Mild	Moderate	Severe
PMS - A								
Nervous Tension	✓				✓			
Mood Swings	✓				✓			
Irritability	✓				✓			
Anxiety	✓				✓			
PMS - H								
*Weight Gain	✓				✓			
Swelling of Extremities	✓				✓			
Breast Tenderness	✓					✓		
Abdominal Bloating	✓				✓			
PMS - C								
Headache	✓				✓			
Craving for Sweets	✓				✓			
Increased Appetite	✓				✓			
Heart Pounding	✓				✓			
Fatigue	✓				✓			
Dizziness or Fainting	✓				✓			
PMS - D								
Depression	✓				✓			
Forgetfulness	✓				✓			
Crying	✓				✓			
Confusion	✓				✓			
Insomnia	✓				✓			
OTHER SYMPTOMS								
Loss of Sexual Interest	✓				✓			
Disorientation	✓				✓			
Clumsiness	✓				✓			
Tremors/Shakes	✓				✓			
Thoughts of Suicide	✓				✓			
Agoraphobia	✓				✓			
Increased Physical Activity	✓				✓			
Heavy/Aching Legs	✓				✓			
Generalized Aches	✓				✓			
Bad Breath	✓				✓			
Sensitivity to Music/Light	✓				✓			
Excessive Thirst	✓				✓			

I was at home for a while and went to the library in desperation taking home eight books on PMS, one of which was Beat PMS Through Diet (the former title of this book), by Maryon Stewart. It seemed from this that I was suffering, amongst other things, from low blood sugar and I needed to get my diet sorted out. Both my doctor and my work colleagues thought that this was logical.

I began eating every three hours to combat feeling faint when I was hungry, but while the symptoms decreased a little they didn't disappear. I contacted the WNAS to get a personal diet plan.

I was put on a special diet and I had to completely reorganize my eating habits. No caffeine, chocolate, refined ugar, sweet things, wheat. I had to eat plenty of fresh fruit and vegetables and increase my exercise regime. I had to take Optivite, Evening Primrose Oil and Normoglycaemia to combat the need for sweet things. I couldn't believe it: feeling better was almost instant and within three months I was absolutely fine. I've got bags of energy. I need less sleep. I go out and do things, like badminton and the gym, and I'm now a sailing instructor. My long-suffering husband is so relieved because he's married to the same person all month! Everything has improved: my self esteem, my ability to function is 100 per cent better and I really feel like I'm in control. Before, I'd have days where I'd feel so angry. Now nothing is a big deal.'

After six months Janet had her PMS well and truly under control. Depression was a phenomenon of the past and her only remaining symptom was slight breast tenderness which has since gone.

The comparison between her two questionnaires clearly shows that her symptoms were attributable to Pre-Menstrual Syndrome and not a psychiatric disorder.

PAULINE'S SUICIDAL FEELINGS

'One day I felt so awful. I had pre-menstrual insomnia and was desperate to get some sleep. I decided I was going to have a good long sleep. I took all the tablets and then after a while I became panic-stricken and chickened out. I called my husband and told him what I'd done. I can't remember much, except he was trying to keep me awake. When the doctor arrived he said, "We've had problems with you threatening to do this before, haven't we? It's your periods isn't it, you always get like that." This was because I'd said I felt like doing it many times in the past.'

9

OTHER SYMPTOMS – CLUMSINESS, LOSS OF SEX DRIVE AND AGORAPHOBIA

After the first year of providing nutritional help to women, it became obvious that there were other pre-menstrual symptoms that were affecting them severely. We made additions to the chart to assess the most common extra symptoms (see chart overleaf).

CLUMSINESS

Clumsiness was the most troublesome additional symptom to our 1,000 patients outside the four sub-groups. Eighty-two per cent of sufferers reported being clumsy pre-menstrually, nearly 58 per cent severe to moderately.

The cause of pre-menstrual clumsiness is uncertain, but it may reflect a disturbance in the finer aspects of nervous system function, which might occur pre-menstrually. This can be caused by changes in brain chemistry, hormonal chemistry, lack of certain nutrients, excessive intake of tea, coffee, cigarettes or alcohol. The presence of pre-menstrual clumsiness suggests that there may well be a substantial physical, rather than psychological, component to such women's pre-menstrual symptoms.

**Degree to which
clumsiness affected a
sample of 1000 women
pre-menstrually**

None	Mild	Moderate	Severe		Total Affected
18%	27%	33%	22%	-	82%

SEX DRIVE

Out of a sample of 1,000 PMS sufferers with sexual relationships 67 per cent reported decreased interest in sex and frequency of sexual intercourse pre-menstrually. Only 1.5 per cent reported increased sexual activity pre-menstrually.

OTHER SYMPTOMS	WEEK BEFORE PERIOD				WEEK AFTER PERIOD			
Loss of Sexual Interest	✓				✓			
Disorientation	✓				✓			
Clumsiness	✓				✓			
Tremors/Shakes	✓				✓			
Thoughts of Suicide	✓				✓			
Agoraphobia	✓				✓			
Increased Physical Activity	✓				✓			
Heavy/Aching Legs	✓				✓			
Generalized Aches	✓				✓			
Bad Breath	✓				✓			
Sensitivity to Music/Light	✓				✓			
Excessive Thirst	✓				✓			

Do you have any other PRE-MENSTRUAL SYMPTOMS not listed above?

1. _____

2. _____

3. _____

4. _____

5. How much weight do you gain before your period? _____

We were concerned to see such a large number of women reporting similar distressing problems, so we decided to follow the progress of a group of 50 severe PMS sufferers, who also had severely decreased sex drive, through a three-month diet and supplement programme to see whether there was any improvement.

After three months these women were asked whether their interest in sex had altered. Fifty per cent of them reported that there had been a complete return to their libido (sex drive) and a further 38 per cent reported a significant but not full improvement to their libido. Only 12 per cent reported no change in libido at all.

The results were obviously very encouraging. Considering neither we nor the women had anticipated improvement in this area initially, it was considered by all to be an added bonus. In most cases the women did not associate their decreased libido with their PMS, and furthermore did not feel that reduced libido was a symptom, but merely a reflection of the state and stage of their relationship. Needless to say, many husbands and partners were satisfied with this particular result.

Improvement in sex drive of 50 women who had previously reported a decrease

Little or no improvement	Significant but not full return to libido	Complete return of libido		Total improvement
12%	38%	50%	-	88%

" Cheryl's Story "

Cheryl Beatty, who suffered as a pre-menstrual chocoholic, and whose story was detailed on page 49, was struggling to maintain her relationship with her husband as her sex drive had all but vanished.

I found the thought of sex irritating

'PMS made me very selfish. I had tunnel vision; I just thought of myself all the time. The suggestion of sex became an irritation and my husband became very long suffering. He knew that sex was off the menu except for one weekend per month if he was lucky.

I am pleased to say that my libido is back and we now have no complaints. The tables are turned and it's me pursuing him. Now it's him who has a headache. We both now enjoy regular sex just as we first did in the days before PMS.

We are far more relaxed. We work together too and there is much more laughter.'

AGORAPHOBIA

On our extended symptom list is the condition of agoraphobia, the exaggerated fear of going out alone. This was eventually added to the list as it seemed to be mentioned far more often than we had anticipated. At about this time we were contacted by a marvellous lady who was running a national group for agoraphobic sufferers. She had some amazing facts and figures about agoraphobia, including statistics on the incidence of PMS-suffering agoraphobic women.

Firstly, we were surprised to learn that 88 per cent of agoraphobia sufferers are women. Out of a sample of 94 agoraphobic women 91 per cent also suffered with PMS!

By coincidence, we had several severe PMS sufferers who also suffered severely with agoraphobia on our programme at this time. Many of them were making excellent progress, not only with the overcoming of their PMS symptoms, but their agoraphobia had also disappeared on the programme.

I'll never forget one joyous phone call I had from a lady in Jersey, who had taken herself out for the day for the first time in eight years. She had gone to have her hair permed and buy some clothes.

As she had previously only gone out accompanied by her husband or a neighbour, when her husband arrived home and found her missing he became understandably worried. After a while he began knocking on neighbours' doors to see whether she had gone visiting. By the time she casually wandered home her husband and neighbours were out in the street looking for her. They couldn't believe her new hair-do, and her husband wasn't sure whether to laugh or cry when he saw how many packages she had! He told me she's been costing him a fortune in evening entertainment ever since! Well, she has got eight years to make up for.

Agoraphobia is a very nasty condition: being afraid to go out is both anti-social and isolating for the victim, and can place an awful strain on a family. Here is the story of a woman who had been perfectly well until she underwent surgery for the purpose of sterilization. The change in her health was so unexpected that it had dramatic repercussions on her life.

66 Hazel's Story 99

Hazel was a 42-year-old mother of three who had been taking anti-depressants for 24 years to ease her agoraphobia and panic attacks. She had little memory of her children when they were small or her part in bringing them up as she had been permanently drugged.

I was like a zombie

'I had my first panic attack when I was 16 following a dental abscess. Looking back, that was the start of my agoraphobia, although I didn't realize it at the time. First of all my doctor put me on iron pills, but when my test came back in the normal range, I was then given tablets for my nerves. I can't remember the name of the first two, but they seemed to make my panic attacks worse. Within a short time I was prescribed Valium – at first 15 mg per day, increasing to 30 mg per day – which I stayed on for 24 years. The Valium knocked me out: I was like a zombie. They seemed to ease the panic attacks initially, but gradually I needed more and more pills to keep the symptoms at bay.

My teenage years were ruined

For the rest of my teenage years my social life was affected as I was unable to go out unaccompanied. I had a boyfriend for a while, but the symptoms of agoraphobia made me afraid to go out and he got fed up waiting around for me. I met my husband at a dance when I was 19. He didn't mind staying in, and we eventually got married when I was 21.

I had our first child when I was 23, and the pregnancy was followed by post-natal depression. I had such severe panic attacks after the birth, every time I went into town, my horizons got smaller until eventually I was housebound and frightened to go through the front door. I couldn't even go

SYMPTOMS

	WEEK AFTER PERIOD (Fill in 3 days after period)				WEEK BEFORE PERIOD (Fill in 2-3 days before period)			
	None	Mild	Moderate	Severe	None	Mild	Moderate	Severe
PMS - A								
Nervous Tension		✓						✓
Mood Swings	✓							✓
Irritability		✓						✓
Anxiety		✓						✓
PMS - H								
*Weight Gain	✓					✓		
Swelling of Extremities	✓							✓
Breast Tenderness	✓							✓
Abdominal Bloating	✓						✓	
PMS - C								
Headache	✓						✓	
Craving for Sweets	✓						✓	
Increased Appetite	✓							✓
Heart Pounding	✓						✓	
Fatigue		✓						✓
Dizziness or Fainting	✓						✓	
PMS - D								
Depression	✓						✓	
Forgetfulness			✓					✓
Crying	✓					✓		
Confusion			✓					✓
Insomnia	✓						✓	
OTHER SYMPTOMS								
Loss of Sexual Interest			✓				✓	
Disorientation	✓						✓	
Clumsiness	✓						✓	
Tremors/Shakes	✓						✓	
Thoughts of Suicide	✓						✓	
Agoraphobia				✓				✓
Increased Physical Activity	✓					✓		
Heavy/Aching Legs	✓						✓	
Generalized Aches	✓						✓	
Bad Breath	✓					✓		
Sensitivity to Music/Light	✓							✓
Excessive Thirst	✓							✓

Do you have any other PRE-MENSTRUAL SYMPTOMS not listed above?

1. _____

2. _____

3. _____

4. _____

*5. How much weight do you gain before your period? __5 lbs__

FOLLOW UP
PRE-MENSTRUAL SYNDROME QUESTIONNAIRE

Name: Hazel _____ Age: 35 _____ Height: _____ Weight: _____

MARITAL STATUS: Single _____ Married _____ Divorced _____ Widowed _____

(Please tick where applicable)

PRESENT CONTRACEPTION: None _____ Pill _____ I.U.D _____ Other _____

  Your periods come every _____ days   Your periods last _____ days

  Your periods are: Light _____   Moderate _____   Heavy _____

SYMPTOMS	WEEK AFTER PERIOD (Fill in 3 days after period)				WEEK BEFORE PERIOD (Fill in 2-3 days before period)			
	None	Mild	Moderate	Severe	None	Mild	Moderate	Severe
PMS - A								
Nervous Tension						✓		
Mood Swings					✓			
Irritability						✓		
Anxiety						✓		
PMS - H								
*Weight Gain					✓			
Swelling of Extremities					✓			
Breast Tenderness					✓			
Abdominal Bloating					✓			
PMS - C								
Headache					✓			
Craving for Sweets					✓			
Increased Appetite					✓			
Heart Pounding					✓			
Fatigue					✓			
Dizziness or Fainting						✓		
PMS - D								
Depression					✓			
Forgetfulness					✓			
Crying					✓			
Confusion					✓			
Insomnia					✓			
OTHER SYMPTOMS								
Loss of Sexual Interest					✓			
Disorientation					✓			
Clumsiness					✓			
Tremors/Shakes					✓			
Thoughts of Suicide					✓			
Agoraphobia						✓		
Increased Physical Activity					✓			
Heavy/Aching Legs					✓			
Generalized Aches					✓			
Bad Breath					✓			
Sensitivity to Music/Light					✓			
Excessive Thirst					✓			

out to do the food shopping. When our son was five he developed cancer in his leg, which I obviously found very stressful. He did survive, thank goodness, but the stress of it left me with obsessional neurosis on top of my agoraphobia. It was a turning point for me. I just sat in a chair all day, didn't bother to cook or clean the house.

I lived on drugs

I eventually had two more children, but I was very afraid during my pregnancies as I felt the Valium might harm the unborn children. I managed to cut down to 20 mg of Valium per day during my pregnancy, but I was too scared to cut down any more as I didn't know how to do without it. I was prescribed a hormone, Duphaston, after the third child, but it did not make any difference.

My husband resorted to working long hours as he couldn't cope with me. Fortunately, the children's school was over the road from our house. I could just about manage to get to the pavement, but I couldn't cross the road as I felt so dizzy. The Valium prescriptions just kept coming. I'd be given 100 pills at a time without ever being seen by the doctor.

After 24 years, in desperation, as my symptoms had become worse before my period was due, I sent my husband out to find a book on PMS, and he came back with Beat PMS Through Diet (the former title of this book). My doctor then offered me beta-blockers and said they weren't habit forming, but I didn't want to take any more drugs. I decided to follow the recommendations in the book and to come off the Valium. I contacted the WNAS and had a telephone consultation.

Coming off Valium was hell. The withdrawal symptoms were like nothing I had ever experienced before. Within six weeks of following the WNAS programme I was feeling human again, and much more like my old self. I even made an appointment to get my hair done. I felt on top of the world. Then I woke up one day feeling really angry and resentful, as I realized I had lost 24 years of my life. I can't even remember the children growing up and I feel so sad about that. My doctor was clearly ignorant, which upsets me greatly, as I can never replace those years.

I have been better for three years now. I am still having some counselling to deal with all the traumas in my life, but the end is in sight. I now cope well with my family and my home, and am getting involved with a local medical charity. Today I am doing the catering for a party of 100 guests to celebrate my father's 90th birthday tomorrow. I couldn't even have dreamt about doing that four years ago! I am so grateful to the WNAS and am trying to persuade them to open a centre in Glasgow as, in my experience, most women don't know that there is help available.'

Although Hazel is very grateful to be well again she is very angry about the lost years in her life. I distinctly remember her phoning me six weeks after she started her programme, expressing her joy that her symptoms had diminished. I was quite surprised to get another phone call a few weeks later from an extremely angry Hazel and at first wondered what had gone wrong. As I sat and listened to her I realized that she was grieving for the years in her life that had passed unnoticed as a result of her medical drug dependency. This story outlines the consequences of a wrong diagnosis, undoubtedly made by someone who had very little knowledge about Pre-Menstrual Syndrome. Despite her anger, for which she has had counselling, Hazel has come to terms with her experience and decided to put it to good use by helping others.

CRIME OR ILLNESS?

Finally in this section, I return to the subject of violence. As violence in general is on the increase in our society I feel this is an area which is certainly worthy of fuller discussion.

As early as 1845 menstrually-related disorders were accepted by the courts as a defence for a criminal act. In that year there were three recorded examples:

- Martha, a servant who, without motive, murdered her employer's child, was acquitted on the grounds of insanity caused by 'obstructed menstruation'.

- A woman was acquitted of murdering her young niece on the grounds of insanity stemming from disordered menstruation.

- A woman servant was accused of theft and was acquitted at Carlisle quarter sessions on the grounds of temporary insanity 'from suppression of the menses'.

So you see, it's not such a new problem. We probably talk openly about it now, whereas years ago it would have been hushed up. More recently there have been other famous cases where PMS has been a large part of the defence.

Dr Dalton reported in *The Lancet* in 1980 the case of a 28-year-old worker in the food industry who was accused of fatally stabbing her girl-friend. Following the stabbing she was admitted to prison and noted to be menstruating. Although she was imprisoned, it was acknowledged that she had severe PMS which was subsequently treated. In 1982 she was freed on probation on the grounds of PMS.

There have been several other similar cases over the past few years. There was the case of Anna Reynolds who battered her mother to death in June 1986. She was convicted of murder in February 1987, and subsequently at appeal the charge was reduced to manslaughter on the basis of diminished responsibility whilst suffering with Pre-Menstrual Syndrome. Debra Lovell was another victim of PMS who became a human fireball after soaking herself in paraffin whilst she was pre-menstrual.

In November 1988 a teenage mother, Donna Kelly, suffering from PMS unintentionally killed her seven-week-old son by shaking him when he would not stop crying. The verdict recorded was not guilty as it was appreciated that Donna Kelly had previously been a loving mother who did not have the intention to kill her baby.

In May 1989 a mother of four killed her son after he 'wound her up'. She walked free from the Old Bailey after the judge said she was sick, rather than evil.

And then there was the case of Nicola Owen who made medical and legal history by becoming the first woman successfully to use PMS as a mitigating plea in the courts, when she was discharged from the Old Bailey where she faced arson charges.

This evidence that some women become more vulnerable, unpredictable and even lose control pre-menstrually and around the time of the onset of their period, confirms the fact that the Pre-Menstrual Syndrome is a common condition which can be life-threatening and should most certainly be taken seriously.

It does, however, mean that PMS may be considered a plausible excuse for an offence. This, I am only too aware, is a very sensitive subject. Like any other scapegoat, it has and will, I'm sure, continue to be used in the courts as a means of reducing or escaping sentence.

Although, at the Women's Nutritional Advisory Service, we have encountered our share of criminal cases, I feel it is important to take a stand on this issue. There is no way that we condone any crime, or believe that a woman should be excused for her actions due to PMS. However, it is acknowledged that PMS can be a contributing factor which should be considered along with all the other factors in each individual case.

Each person, be they male or female, has the responsibility to look after their own body. There is evidence now, for example, that indicates that poor diet is related to delinquency and even dyslexia.

Rather than excusing women with PMS for their actions, or adolescents who offend for their behaviour, it would be better to help them overcome the problem by at least correcting their nutritional state. The upsetting and frustrating fact is that much education is needed, both for the public and also for the medical profession. Just knowing which foods help and which foods may harm would be a great start. Having some basic understanding of how diet can affect one's state of mind, for instance, would be invaluable.

We hope that over the next few years doctors will be taking all this into consideration, much more so than they are generally doing at present.

In the meantime, the courts have the difficult task of deciding where to draw the line. There should certainly be the facility for them to check on a woman's nutritional state and have her assessed for PMS. This assessment usually would take three months to confirm as three consecutive cycles need to be charted in order to confirm the diagnosis of PMS.

The fact that a woman may be a danger to herself or society has to be dealt with in a routine way by the courts. When PMS is presented as a defence or mitigation, and the diagnosis confirmed, then effective treatment should be sought whilst the woman is serving her sentence, if she has been convicted.

It is very important that when PMS is used as a defence or mitigation, appropriate treatment is instituted. It then becomes the woman's personal responsibility to follow the appropriate diet or take the appropriate treatment to ensure that her pre-menstrual symptoms are properly controlled. PMS could then not be used as a defence or mitigation should she then re-offend.

10

THE SOCIAL IMPLICATIONS OF PMS

RELATIONSHIPS AT HOME AND AT WORK

It was not surprising that as a result of these severe symptoms, we were recording that some of our survey of women reported that their home lives and relationships with family and friends were affected by their PMS symptoms.

Degree to which a sample of 1000 women felt that their home life/relationship with family/friends was affected due to PMS symptoms

Not Affected	Mild	Moderate	Severe		Total Affected
5%	9%	30%	56%	-	95%

You will have read in earlier sections about how some family lives were affected. I have added two quite different examples here to make the point in its own right, as the family and our immediate circle are so very important.

Marcia is a 16-year-old schoolgirl who displayed antisocial characteristics before her period. She had been caught in a PMS trap for four years, since her periods began at the time when she contacted the WNAS.

'My symptoms were severe and lasted for about 18 days each month before my period was due. In fact, one month I even contemplated ending my life as it didn't seem worth living. I used to feel utterly antisocial and incredibly tired, just wanting to sleep all the time. I had extreme cravings for sweet foods and could easily eat six chocolate bars in one sitting followed by masses of cakes and biscuits. I would stuff myself with all the sweet food I could lay my hands on until I was almost unconscious.

I also experienced terrible period pains which sent me to bed each month for at least seven to ten days. When I approached the WNAS I was pretty desperate as I was in the middle of doing my GCSEs.

I felt so aggressive

My mother and I normally get on reasonably well but our relationship went to seed pre-menstrually. I could feel the aggression welling within me and I knew I wouldn't rest until we had had a full-blown argument. My mother didn't believe I had period problems and thought I was skiving off school. The shouting matches between us always ended in me saying the most horrible things which I didn't mean. I felt utterly ashamed afterwards.

My doctor suggested I take vitamin B6 and painkillers to help ease the period pain. I was really desperate to find some help and fortunately read about the work of the WNAS. I contacted them and enrolled in their telephone consultation service. I was given explicit advice about what to eat and drink and in particular what to avoid in the short term. I hadn't been doing much exercise and so I was asked to build up gradually to four sessions a week, and to take some vitamins and minerals.

Within a month of beginning my programme I was feeling considerably better and within two months I had no symptoms whatsoever. I got through my GCSEs and did well which I didn't dream would happen. I then managed to get myself a full-time job with day release so that I could continue at college, and am honestly feeling brilliant. At first I thought my symptoms might return but it has been eight months now and I still have absolutely no symptoms. I have made things up with my mother and she now understands that my symptoms were related to my periods. Relationships at home have calmed down considerably and are happy and enjoyable.'

Marcia's undoing came about as a result of her continually eating masses of chocolate, cakes and biscuits, instead of healthy food. Her recovery was rapid once she was on a normal healthy diet and exercise regime. Marcia now feels that she is able to lead a normal life on every day of her cycle without having to live in fear of her period approaching.

PERSONAL RELATIONSHIPS

It is exceedingly difficult to maintain a loving relationship when you are experiencing severe symptoms of irritability, nervous tension and aggression. I so often see women whose personal and sexual relationships have fallen apart as a direct result of their PMS. Judy and Liz are two good examples of how symptoms stood in the way of a harmonious personal life. The good news is that they both, like the majority of our patients, were able to restore their relationships once over their symptoms. It is not uncommon for men to thank us for giving them back the girl they married!

❝ Judy's Story ❞

Judy was a 44-year-old mother with three children, the eldest of whom was 15. She had suffered from PMS since the birth of her second child in 1984.

'I had suffered with terrible depression and mood swings. I'd feel fuzzy in the head and cry a lot, feeling that I couldn't cope with things. I had insomnia really badly and most of the time I felt negative about everything. Sometimes I would crave chocolates, packets of biscuits and crisps when I felt depressed, which was usually three out of four weeks. I felt good when I'd had them and then felt terrible for succumbing. I had constipation too, for as long as I can remember, which led to me feeling bloated and fat. Life was all doom and gloom.

I was being counselled by a clinical psychologist on a six-weekly basis for about two years which didn't result in anything positive. I asked my gynaecologist to find out about hormone imbalance but all he did was put me on HRT which didn't improve my condition at all. My GP arranged for me to attend a psychiatrist on his suggestion, and I had two meetings but felt it was a total waste of time.

I preferred the cat to my husband

All this affected my husband very badly. I never seemed to have much sexual desire for him since my third child. I was always too tired and ready to just take a sleeping pill and curl up on my bed with the cat. I'd be verbally abusive and appeared to be unable to show him any affection. He'd touch me and I'd back off. I couldn't respond to any affection which eventually led to no sex at all between us. We slept in separate bedrooms. Many times I wanted to go to him and would stand outside his door but couldn't quite manage it. I made myself drunk one night so that I might get some attention from him. I wanted him to notice me, I suppose.

Fat and worthless

I was so unreasonable with the children, nagging them about everything they did. In the end they didn't offer any help in the house because the work wouldn't be up to my expectations. Although I gave up full-time work when the children came along, I found it hard to accept the loss of independence. I had had a very fulfilling career and a very pressured job. I'd had several different part-time jobs but I found I had lost my confidence and assertiveness. In the last three years I had gained three stones in weight and felt really bad about myself. I didn't have the strength to go to Weight Watchers or to help myself.

My husband left me

Early in 1996 my husband moved out. He was really stressed and depressed with me, was pressured at work and we had financial troubles. I was desperate.'

Judy was in a very low state when I first met up with her. She had terrible panic attacks and insomnia, and at the age of 44 was utterly bewildered about how she would cope with her three children, the eldest of whom was 15, in the absence of her husband. She had suffered with PMS since the birth of her second child in 1984.

'A friend suggested I get the book Beat PMS Through Diet by Maryon Stewart of the WNAS. As soon as I started reading it everything fell into place. Ten days later I had my first consultation with Maryon. She advised me to go on a gluten-free diet, exclude caffeine, eat plenty of fresh fish, fruit and vegetables and to increase my exercise regime. It was suggested I should take magnesium to keep my bowels open on a daily basis – this had never been known! I also took Optivite and Normoglycaemia. I felt some of the

JUDY

SYMPTOMS	WEEK AFTER PERIOD (Fill in 3 days after period)				WEEK BEFORE PERIOD (Fill in 2-3 days before period)			
	None	Mild	Moderate	Severe	None	Mild	Moderate	Severe
PMS - A								
Nervous Tension		✓						✓
Mood Swings		✓						✓
Irritability	✓						✓	
Anxiety		✓						✓
PMS - H								
*Weight Gain	✓					✓		
Swelling of Extremities	✓				✓			
Breast Tenderness	✓				✓			
Abdominal Bloating	✓						✓	
PMS - C								
Headache	✓				✓			
Craving for Sweets	✓						✓	
Increased Appetite	✓					✓		
Heart Pounding	✓					✓		
Fatigue		✓					✓	
Dizziness or Fainting	✓				✓			
PMS - D								
Depression			✓					✓
Forgetfulness	✓						✓	
Crying		✓						✓
Confusion		✓				✓		
Insomnia			✓					✓
OTHER SYMPTOMS								
Loss of Sexual Interest	✓						✓	
Disorientation	✓					✓		
Clumsiness	✓						✓	
Tremors/Shakes	✓					✓		
Thoughts of Suicide	✓					✓		
Agoraphobia	✓					✓		
Increased Physical Activity		✓			✓			
Heavy/Aching Legs	✓				✓			
Generalized Aches	✓				✓			
Bad Breath	✓				✓			
Sensitivity to Music/Light	✓				✓			
Excessive Thirst	✓					✓		

Do you have any other PRE-MENSTRUAL SYMPTOMS not listed above?

1. Fluid retention – before period 2-3 days.

2. Onset of period – I have to go to pass urine more frequently than

3. usual – cannot hold it in bladder as long

4.

*5. How much weight do you gain before your period? 2-4 lbs approx

FOLLOW UP
PRE-MENSTRUAL SYNDROME QUESTIONNAIRE

Name: Judy   Age: 45   Height: 5' 5"   Weight: 11st 7lb

MARITAL STATUS: Single _____ Married _____ Divorced _____ Widowed _____
(Please tick where applicable)

PRESENT CONTRACEPTION: None _____ Pill _____ I.U.D _____ Other _____

   Your periods come every _____ days   Your periods last _____ days

   Your periods are: Light _____   Moderate ✓   Heavy ✓

SYMPTOMS	WEEK AFTER PERIOD (Fill in 3 days after period)				WEEK BEFORE PERIOD (Fill in 2-3 days before period)			
	None	Mild	Moderate	Severe	None	Mild	Moderate	Severe
PMS - A								
Nervous Tension	✓				✓			
Mood Swings	✓				✓			
Irritability	✓				✓			
Anxiety	✓				✓			
PMS - H								
*Weight Gain	✓					✓		
Swelling of Extremities	✓				✓			
Breast Tenderness	✓				✓			
Abdominal Bloating	✓				✓			
PMS - C								
Headache	✓				✓			
Craving for Sweets	✓				✓			
Increased Appetite	✓				✓			
Heart Pounding	✓					✓		
Fatigue	✓				✓			
Dizziness or Fainting	✓				✓			
PMS - D								
Depression	✓				✓			
Forgetfulness	✓				✓			
Crying	✓				✓			
Confusion	✓				✓			
Insomnia	✓					✓		
OTHER SYMPTOMS								
Loss of Sexual Interest	✓				✓			
Disorientation	✓				✓			
Clumsiness	✓				✓			
Tremors/Shakes	✓				✓			
Thoughts of Suicide	✓				✓			
Agoraphobia	✓				✓			
Increased Physical Activity	✓				✓			
Heavy/Aching Legs	✓				✓			
Generalized Aches	✓				✓			
Bad Breath	✓				✓			
Sensitivity to Music/Light	✓				✓			
Excessive Thirst	✓				✓			

symptoms, such as the constipation, easing in the first month. It is almost nine months now and I feel so much better. My life has been transformed. I feel positive about myself and try not to let anything get me down; I'm so relaxed. My husband is back home now and I am so happy. PMS disrupted my family life. Everything seemed like an impossible hurdle to get over. Sometimes I didn't want to associate with my friends, my sister or my parents. My husband left me because I rejected him. It felt like he didn't know what I was going through or how bad I felt.

Now I realize that my husband and children needed to be wanted too. The change in my diet and lifestyle has been my lifesaver. I am much calmer with the children and don't lose my patience with them if something goes wrong. I don't shout and scream at them as I used to. I really don't feel as if I'm in a rut any more and the programme has resulted in the return of the real "me".'

Judy's story is an example of how close many PMS sufferers come to losing a potentially good relationship. What was overwhelmingly clear at her first appointment was that she desperately loved her husband but because of her symptoms and lack of clarity, thought she had almost pushed him to the point of no return. Over the years we have seen many patients in this state, some of whom regularly visit their solicitor once a month to initiate divorce proceedings. Women often express irrational feelings of hate for their partner in their pre-menstrual phase which miraculously fade away with the onset of a period. Overcoming symptoms of PMS opens the door to the possibility of resurrecting some of the most broken-down relationships you can imagine. The letter from Judy's husband, who is a quiet, retiring individual, sums up the frustration that men often feel watching their partners suffer.

Recently I saw a patient in the clinic who was told by her husband to tell me that he felt that there was a third person in their marriage. When she came for her follow-up appointment she brought with her another message from her husband informing me that the third person had moved out.

Dear Maryon,

You will remember how desperate I was for help when you kindly saw me in May of 1996. My husband had had enough of me and the situation I was in, and he had to get out to keep himself from 'cracking up'.

You know what alternatives I had tried without any positive result. To me, you are my lifesaver, you have found the root of my problem, you have helped me tremendously to find myself again. I don't have the awful depression and crying and mood swings to put up with. you put me straight on the magnesium to give me a regular bowel movement! Being constipated made me miserable/bloated/uncomfortable/and liverish as you know.

I no longer dread the thought of the 'bad days' coming. Sometimes my period kind of 'taps me on the shoulder' from nowhere. My diet programme, wheat free, was to play a major role in sorting me out, together with Optivite. I never take anything for granted any more, and I'm so grateful I feel well again, with my husband back and a normal family life.

Judy Harrington

Dear Maryon,

As I am quite a 'laid-back' person, when after our second child my wife became moody, tearful and depressed, I thought that after a short while she would get over it.

But as time went by I found the problems got worse. We tried conventional remedies (doctor, gynaecologist, anti-depressants, HRT, sleeping pills, etc.) but the symptoms remained.

As I did not understand (or know) about this PMS problem, I began to switch off to the situation. In the end I left my wife for two and a half months. In this time my wife had heard about the WNAS and contacted you.

When I came to visit the family, I found the change in her remarkable. Over a short period of time she had calmed down and was reverting back to the woman that I once knew and loved. We found we could talk more freely about PMS and other problems.

But most of all we found our love again.

Robert Harrington

PRODUCTIVITY AND EFFICIENCY AT WORK

Another incredible statistic that emerged from the study on 1000 PMS sufferers was the degree to which their work suffered as a result of their symptoms. 83 per cent reported that their productivity and efficiency decreased pre-menstrually.

They further reported that they were, to a large degree, 'not there mentally' for an average of five days per month! This means that they produce very little work during this period of time.

66 Iona's Story 99

Iona is a 29-year-old barrister who suffered with PMS for 17 years.

'My worst PMS symptoms were nausea. I always felt nausea and in the latter years I would be continuously vomiting, which I found the hardest thing to deal with. Apart from that I used to feel very depressed. I'd be very weepy, upset and emotional for no apparent reason. I used to put on weight and become very bloated.

PMS affected my work

I always felt I wasn't functioning properly and wasn't doing my best workwise. I'm a barrister and I need to be able to concentrate and I need to be able to think very quickly, but when I was suffering from my symptoms, I wasn't able to do that and consequently it affected my work. I'd always hope that when my symptoms came I had a case that was easy to deal with and didn't involve a lot of work or concentration.

Altogether I had suffered with PMS for 17 years. I had been to several gynaecologists to get help with my symptoms. Initially my GP had told me that I would continue to have these symptoms until I had my first child; since I started my period when I was 11 that wasn't very helpful. I was put on the pill at the age of 16 and I took the pill for 10 years to deal with the symptoms; but it wasn't very helpful. It was only helpful in so much as it would suppress symptoms during exam times.

My symptoms vanished overnight

When I went on the PMS programme I was told I would have to cut out chocolate from my diet, which I found very hard because I love chocolate. Also I was told to avoid foods containing wheat and alcohol before my symptoms arrived, to exercise and to take the recommended supplements. Having done that for a month, and I stuck regularly to the programme, my symptoms just vanished overnight. It was just absolutely amazing. Normally the symptoms would be there, but I had no symptoms whatsoever, it was an answer to a prayer, and after 17 years of suffering it was just brilliant!'

A labour force survey conducted in 1996 found that there were just over 11.5 million working women in the UK. Over 10.7 million were employed and the remainder were self-employed. Given these figures the cost to industry due to lack of production must be vast, and probably not a statistic that has been properly considered. It wouldn't register as sickness or absenteeism as these women appear to be at work in the normal way. Unless specifically asked for, this information would not appear. Indeed, even asking for it may not produce the truth as there are so many women who would be in fear of losing their jobs. As it is, they feel they are teetering on the edge of disaster at work because of their general behaviour pre-menstrually. **81.6 per cent** of 1,000 women felt that their work or career had been adversely affected by their PMS. So keeping a low profile is the least line of resistance.

Effects on productivity/efficiency pre-menstrually out of a sample of 1000 women

Same	Decreased	Increased
17%	83%	0%

In 1993 the results of a study we undertook on work efficiency were published. It was to my knowledge the first study of its kind in the UK. In conjunction with Kimberly-Clark, the makers of Kleenex and Simplicity products, we were able to work with 47 of their staff who were suffering with PMS. The group was split into two, with half the women making dietary changes and taking Optivite, and the other half just making dietary changes. There was an improvement in work efficiency in both groups with a trend towards increased benefit in the group taking the nutritional supplement as well. As a group all the women reported an increased sense of well-being and energy levels.

A look at case histories of women who came to the Women's Nutritional Advisory Service proves the point. There was Frankie Ferguson, a single parent, who worked as a Human Resources officer.

66 Frankie's Story 99

'I had suffered with PMS for some time but my symptoms became particularly bad after the birth of my son and the breakup of my relationship. For the week or sometimes two before my period it felt like my brain was gone. I would be very aggressive with my son, less tolerant of mistakes he made than I would be normally and at work my customers and colleagues were treated with far less patience and tolerance.

I felt that I was wasting two weeks every month, particularly at work as my productivity and creativity were at an all-time low. I would want to sleep more and hide away in the evenings of those two weeks. I read about the

*work of the WNAS in ME magazine and approached them for help. I
followed their recommendations as closely as I could and started going to
exercise classes with my sister. Gradually things started to improve. My cycle
went from being 26 days to a regular 30-day cycle with no cycle dribs and
drabs, which was great in itself. The fatigue lifted and I began to feel calmer
and more in control.*

*I began my programme 12 months ago and I can honestly say I feel so
earthed now, so laid back I could almost fall over. Life at home with my son
is normal again and I am managing far better at work. My colleagues have
noticed that there has been a big change and, in fact, I have recently won an
award out of all employees. It is the first time our company has run this
scheme in its present form so I was particularly pleased to be chosen. I
received a cheque for £250 and a bottle of champagne but the best gift of all
was that I have found myself again.'*

It obviously wasn't only Frankie's friends and family who noticed a
dramatic change in her behaviour and performance as a result of overcoming her PMS symptoms. She is much more confident these days and really
chuffed by this award.

You may remember Maureen's story on page 32. She was fighting for sur-
vival at work and at the time she approached the WNAS was being
screened by occupational health with a view to some sort of drastic action
due to her lack of performance. She used to struggle to look after 30 staff
members and was often absent from work.

❝ Maureen's Story ❞

*'Within three months of following the WNAS programme I had lost half a
stone in weight, I was wonderfully stable each day and had regained my
enthusiasm for life. I had renewed my friendships, applied to do an MA in
education which had been a goal I never dared hope for, and within one
month was promoted to co-ordinator at work. It has now been two years
since my treatment with the WNAS and I even manage to cope well with my
stressful job. These days I am responsible for 150 students. I won the
hospital contract to train qualified staff nurses to be NVQ assessors. I am
actively involved in training and research and have managed to develop a
successful research package which is now being implemented in our local
area. Considering not so many years ago I was lurching from one day to the
next not knowing what the future holds I am extremely hoppy with the
outcome.'*

You will have come across Gail's story on page 53. She spent so much time eating chocolate and feeling ill as a result that she was quite unable to hold down a job. Following her programme at the WNAS she has re-trained and become a partner in an estate agency firm.

❝ Gail's Story ❞

'I'd raid the house for anything chocolatey. And if I couldn't find anything my poor husband would have to go and get me my "fix". I'd even raid the children's chocolate box. This went on for 21 days out of my 28-day cycle. I put on so much weight and experienced feelings of violence and aggression which were vented at my family for no apparent reason. During my one clear week I'd tell myself that the next time it would be different, but of course a week later I was that madwoman all over again: cramming my face with chocolate and hating myself for it.

I visted my GP and was told my bingeing symptoms were psychosomatic. He prescribed the pill for my heavy periods and sent me off. Initially this did the trick and my periods lightened, but there was a major drawback. The listlessness, bingeing and low feelings got much worse on the pill so after a couple of months I stopped taking it which meant of course that I was back to square one.

The turning point came when I read a magazine article about a woman who had suffered the problems I was experiencing. I immediately contacted the WNAS which was featured in the piece. With their guidance I gave up chocolate and caffeine, wheat and dairy products. Amazingly, within a few months I was completely back to normal. My cravings disappeared and I began losing weight. All my pre-menstrual symptoms were gone and my periods became light. It is five years now and I've never looked back. I am a totally different person, and I cannot stress enough that the person suffering with PMS was not me at all. Then, I was unable to cope with a job, and now I have retrained as an estate agent and become a partner! I enjoy a normal family life and my children no longer regard me as a time bomb. The WNAS literally saved me and gave me back my life.'

DRIVING ABILITY

Many of the symptoms discussed have broad repercussions on the sufferer herself and on her family and friends. However, the seriousness of PMS comes right home when a statistic appears that could affect us all. We asked 1000 drivers who suffer with PMS whether their driving ability was affected pre-menstrually. An astounding **76.9 per cent** said their driving ability decreased before their period. Many women stop driving before their period is due as they have previously had so many accidents pre-menstrually. The two main factors that seem to affect driving ability are lack of concentration and poor coordination. Amazingly, the women report that as soon as their period arrives, their driving ability returns to normal.

Driving a car, or any vehicle for that matter, is a real responsibility and not to be taken lightly. We advise severe sufferers to keep off the road until their symptoms have gone, or are under control. Placing lives at risk is no joke. Here are two examples of many who experienced diminished driving skills pre-menstrually.

❝ Natasha's Story ❞

'My inability to cope was apparent in other things too. Through lack of co-ordination I pranged the car when parking and dented my bumper – nothing serious thank goodness. I was so forgetful I left the car window open all night – it rained. Another time I left the sunroof open all night – it poured. I drove through red traffic lights, and once I packed the children and the shopping into the car and left the buggy behind when I drove off.'

❝ Clare's Story ❞

'I was unable to concentrate and had two car accidents when I was pre-menstrual. The first was when I pulled away from the kerb and struck another car that was on the opposite side of the road. Suddenly my co-ordination had gone and I had become really disorientated: I couldn't even remember where my brake pedal was and I couldn't stop. It was an awful experience. The second time I slowly reversed into another parked car. After that I wouldn't drive at all for two days before my period for my own and others' safety.'

PART TWO

NUTRITION AND
OUR BODIES

11

WHY IS PMS MORE COMMON TODAY?

As I have already mentioned, PMS seems to be more common today than in years past. This is undoubtedly partly because it is talked about now in a way that was inconceivable 30 or 40 years ago. But it is probably also due to changes in our lifestyle, diet and possibly our use of hormones and drugs. It is extremely hard to pinpoint any one factor as being a clear-cut cause of PMS. But though the case may not be proven, it may be useful to look at some of these factors and their relationship with PMS and other common diseases that have become the hallmark of the twentieth century.

It is estimated that in 1993 the NHS bill for the taxpayer was £41 billion. In the USA in the last 20 or so years, the medical bill has increased from $27 billion to over $400 billion (1996 figures)! The awful fact is that, despite these amounts of money being spent, some of us have been getting sicker.

Cardiovascular disease is still the biggest killer in developed countries and undoubtedly the commonest preventable cause of early death in young to middle-aged men and women. Approximately 300,000 people die each year in the United Kingdom from heart attacks and strokes. There has been little improvement, as yet, in these figures, though the United States and Finland have begun to achieve a substantial fall in their incidences of heart disease. Smoking, lack of exercise, obesity, high blood pressure and high blood cholesterol are all well-documented risk factors and these last three are all influenced by diet.

Cancer too, it appears, is on the increase. There seem to be three main factors for this. The first is age. With a few exceptions the incidence of most cancers rises steeply with age from about 40 years onward. In times past many people did not live long enough to be at risk of developing cancer. Secondly, it is highly likely that there has been a true increase in the rate of cancer this century, regardless of age, and that this reflects the increased use of chemicals in the environment. Many industrial chemicals, pesticides and even drugs linger in the environment for years. Finally, the type of food we eat also influences cancer risk. Consumption of smoked and pickled foods is associated with an increase in some cancers, especially of the stomach and oesophagus, whilst a high intake of fresh fruit and vegetables may well protect against many types of cancer. These protective foods are rich in vitamin C, E and carotene – vegetable vitamin A – which help limit the damage to tissues by cancer-inducing chemicals.

'Mental' illnesses are also on the increase and this too may be influenced by our diet, consumption of alcohol, medical and illicit drugs. Obviously social factors, education and life skills are also all important in helping us cope with times of stress or ill-health. The stresses and strains of twentieth-century living have not made it easy for some of us to cope, and for many women, working and raising a family is particularly stressful.

Allergic problems have also become much more common in the last 40 years. The reasons for this are not clear but include family or genetic factors, chemicals in the environment, dietary habits and the pattern of feeding in childhood.

What, I hear you ask, has this pessimistic view of the state of our health got to do with PMS? Quite simply, it appears that the development of PMS is very much influenced by the same factors: diet, exercise or lack of it, and possibly environmental chemicals. It is possible that these diverse conditions have common causative and aggravating factors.

In 1986 the Women's Nutritional Advisory Service completed a national street survey on 500 women in Britain. We found that 73.6 per cent of them suffered in varying degrees with PMS. This figure is considerably more than estimates of 30–60 per cent made during the previous 30 years.

By now you must be wondering why the diseases are becoming more common, and you might well ask. Our twentieth-century lifestyle brings many relatively new experiences to us, some of which we are not well equipped to handle. The diets most of us know are very far removed from those of our ancestors. Our bodies were not built to cope with refined and processed foods, very often empty of nutrients. We have had to live with pesticides and insecticides being sprayed on our crops, growth hormones and antibiotics pumped into animals, and environmental pollution and acid rain as the finishing touches. Many of us over-eat and under-exercise, and women nowadays tend to lead far more stressful existences. So it is logical, really, that we can't honestly expect our 'machines' to go on indefinitely without breaking down when we don't treat them with respect. We generally treat our cars better than we do our bodies – you wouldn't dream of putting the wrong fuel in your petrol tank, would you?

Before I launch into the tale of woe about our diet, let me say that although you will probably come to realize that we are faced with certain problems concerning our diet, with good education we *can* find ways around them. I will of course be discussing various solutions in the Self-Help section on diet in Part Three.

A GOOD LOOK AT OUR DIET

In order to look at diet more closely we need to examine how our habits have changed during this century.

- We have increased our consumption of sugar. The UK has become one of the world's largest chocolate and sweet eaters, with the average person consuming some 130 pounds or 12.7 kilos each per year. We currently spend over £3.2 billion per year on chocolate alone.

- Our diet is particularly high in saturated fats (animal fats). It is thought that this has much to do with our also having a high incidence of heart disease and breast cancer.

- We eat far too much salt – 10 to 20 times more than our bodies really require per day. Salt can contribute to blood pressure problems and pre-menstrual water retention.

- We often drink far too much coffee and tea which can impede the absorption of essential nutrients. On average we consume four cups of tea and two cups of coffee per day, but many people exceed this.

- We consume volumes of foods with a high level of phosphorus, which again impedes absorption of good nutrients. Examples of these foods are soft drinks of low or normal calorie types, processed foods, canned, packaged, pre-packed, convenience foods and ready-made sauces.

- Alcohol consumption has almost doubled in the United Kingdom since the end of the Second World War. On average, women drink about the equivalent of one unit per day (equal to one glass of wine). Not much, you may think, but enough to have a slight adverse effect on the outcome of pregnancy! Also, about one-third of women are teetotal or consume very little alcohol so someone is having their share.

- Unbelievable as it may seem, we actually eat less food than we did thirty and more years ago. It seems that women of today actually expend less energy than those of a generation or two ago and this has resulted in a 10 to 15 per cent reduction in food intake. This means that our intake of essential nutrients has also fallen, particularly if we eat refined or convenience foods. The motor car and lack of exercise has almost certainly been a factor in the decline in energy expenditure.

- Many of the foods available contain chemical additives in the form of flavour enhancers, colouring and preservatives. Whilst some of these are not harmful, some of them *are*, and our bodies are certainly not designed to cope with them.

- In many areas our water contains certain pollutants which are thought to be a risk to public health.

- Our meat has become contaminated with antibiotics and growth hormones, and with the advent of mad cow disease it can sometimes kill us off.

- Nitrate fertilizers have been used to obtain fast-growing and abundant crops. It is now recognized that nitrates are harmful and can produce cancer, at least in animals.

- Almost all of our fresh fruit, cereals and vegetables are sprayed with pesticides at least once. In addition, milk and meat may retain the pesticides from feed given to livestock.

Smoking

Smoking tobacco has become a widespread habit among Western societies. In 1922 in the United Kingdom, for example, 20–34-year-old women smoked an average of 50 cigarettes per year, but by 1994 this had risen to an average of just over 5,000 cigarettes per woman, per year. Despite the more educated classes reducing their cigarette consumption, smoking has become relatively more common amongst women, in those who are less well educated.

Alcohol

Since the 1940s alcohol consumption has doubled in the United Kingdom. On average, women consume one unit of alcohol per day, and men three units (one unit =1 glass of wine, 1 pub measure of spirits, 1 small sherry or vermouth, or half a pint of normal strength beer or lager). These average levels are now the maximum recommended daily intakes for women and men respectively. Whilst many of us may be teetotallers, or drink substantially less than this, there will be those who regularly consume more. Some women may go on pre-menstrual alcohol binges.

Twenty-five per cent of our weekly spend is on alcohol and tobacco. Just think how the quality of our diet would improve if we reduced this percentage.

Drugs

Western societies have become drug-oriented. In the 12 months of 1996 in the United States nearly £72 billion was spent on medicines by a population of 266 million, and in the UK it was £5.5 billion or £100 per man/woman and child. Doctors issue some 15 per cent more prescriptions than they did a decade ago. In England only, over 425 million prescriptions were written in 1992, nearly 10 million for anti-depressants, amounting to £81 million. Not surprising in view of the power and influence that drug companies have been allowed to assume in the education of doctors.

In the last year there has been tremendous concern by medical practitioners worldwide about the excessive use of benzodiazepene tranquillizers and sleeping tablets. It is now recommended that these drugs, which include Valium, Mogadon and Ativan, are used as a temporary measure for only a few weeks. Those who have been taking them long-term should, if at all possible, have their dosage and frequency gradually reduced under medical supervision.

The Pill

The oral contraceptive birth control pill has been a popular and effective method of contraception. The initial forms of the birth pill had large amounts of oestrogen, which were known to cause some disturbance in vitamin and mineral balance, increase the risk of vaginal thrush, and in some women precipitate significant depression and migraine headaches. These side-effects are less likely with the new lower dose, or phased dosage oral contraceptive pill. However, problems can certainly arise. Whilst the oral contraceptive pill can help some women's pre-menstrual symptoms, and is a useful way for treating mild PMS, particularly in those women who require contraception, it can also aggravate some PMS symptoms. There is no way of determining this, other than by trial and error. If you find an oral contraceptive pill that suits you, all well and good. However, some women will find that practically any form of the Pill aggravates their pre-menstrual symptoms.

Vitamin and mineral intake

Our diet this century has gone through, and continues to go through, several substantial changes. By the end of the 1970s there was evidence, from certain surveys, of a deterioration in the quality of the UK diet, particularly since the Second World War. A high intake of sugar, refined foods, animal fats and alcohol had meant a relatively poor intake of essential vitamins and minerals.

Some fifteen vitamins, twenty-four minerals and eight amino acids have been isolated as being essential for normal body function. They are synergistic, which means that they rely upon each other in order to keep the body functioning at an optimum level. When one or more is in short supply, alterations in body metabolism occur. Minor deficiencies can often be tolerated, but major or multiple deficiencies result in the body becoming inefficient, with the development of symptoms and possibly disease.

There is, however, some heartening recent evidence. All the good advice from numerous individual experts and expert committees, government ones included, has finally got through to *some* of the British public. Many of us have increased our intake of fruit and vegetables and this greatly offsets the potential fall in intake from eating refined foods or eating smaller amounts of food in general. However, this has not happened with the unemployed or those who come from families where the main wage-earner is unskilled. From the recent dietary survey of British adults in the UK, the single biggest factor that determined nutrient intake was not age, sex, illness, or whether on a diet or not, but whether the person was unemployed. Like it or not, it seems that we already have a nutritional underclass who don't have the money and the knowledge to improve their diets. Fats and sugar are cheap calories, and when you are hungry calories are more important than fibre or vitamins and minerals.

Let us now turn our attention to certain specific nutrients which may contribute to symptoms of PMS.

THE NITTY GRITTY REVIEW
OF SPECIFIC NUTRIENTS

Some nutritional factors may be of particular importance to PMS. In the United Kingdom, the Department of Health has instructed the Committee on the Medical Aspects of Food to investigate the nature of the UK diet, and what the appropriate intakes of calories, fats, fibre, vitamins and minerals should be. A similar governmental review by the Food and Drug Administration in the USA was also undertaken in the 1980s.

In 1991 the Department of Health in the UK published its report on Dietary Reference Values for Food Energy and Nutrients for the United Kingdom. This report was prepared by an august group of scientists and doctors who set guidelines for intakes for most of the known essential nutrients. It followed another important report, The Dietary and Nutritional Survey of British Adults. These two reports and similar reports from the United States have allowed a more detailed assessment than ever before of the nutritional adequacy for the adult population in these two developed countries.

Vitamin B

The B group of vitamins, and in particular vitamin B6, have been used for many years to treat PMS. In the UK the new recommended average intake for women of child-bearing age is 1.2 mg per day, exactly the level found in an independent nutrition survey (the Booker Health Report 1985) and less than the value of 1.7 mg from the recent government survey. According to these figures, hardly anyone should be deficient in this nutrient. But several surveys using blood tests have revealed that some 10 to 20 per cent of adults, especially women, appear to have a mild deficiency. This seems more likely in those with problems such as depression and anxiety, as well as PMS. However, deficiency of this nutrient does not explain PMS as many of those with a mild deficiency have no symptoms at all.

Folic acid, another of the B vitamins, was found to be slightly low in between 8 and 40 per cent of adult women. Young women seemed particularly at risk. These figures are almost certainly an overestimate of the problem and comparable surveys from the US give values less than half these, but still with no cause for complacency.

Deficiency of these two B group vitamins and the others (B1, B2, B3 and B12), which occur less frequently, can all affect energy level, mood, skin quality, hormone function and appetite. A poor intake may contribute in part to some women's PMS. Certain aspects of our modern diet deserve further comment.

Many refined foods are low in B complex vitamins. For example, a McDonald's Big Mac hamburger is known to contain only a fraction of the vitamin B6 that it should do. Presumably, substantial quantities are lost in preparation, cooking and storage. In fact, you would have to eat 60 Big Mac hamburgers a day, in order to achieve an intake of 1.2 mg of vitamin B6 – a current conservative allowance.

Thus, for some of us whose diets do not contain good quantities of fresh and wholesome foods, the intake of B vitamins may be low.

Magnesium

Magnesium is a key mineral in the treatment of PMS. It has now been shown in several medical studies that women with PMS have low levels of magnesium in their red blood cells, and finding a mildly reduced level of magnesium in the blood is now the most consistent reported abnormal finding in women with PMS. Once again, however, not all women with a low level of blood magnesium will have PMS.

Intakes of this mineral in the UK are generally below optimum levels: aproximately 15 per cent of all women in the UK of child-bearing age eat a diet deficient in magnesium, and many others consume only borderline amounts – a low intake (i.e. likely to lead to deficiency) has been defined in the UK as less than 150 mg per day; the recommended intakes and actual intakes in the United States are higher but without any cause for complacency. It may come as no surprise to you to learn that vegetables, fruit and all unrefined or unprocessed foods are rich in this mineral and that refined foods are poor sources. Eating a diet low in protein and high in salt, sugar, alcohol and possibly coffee may contribute to increased losses of magnesium. Like the B vitamins, magnesium has an effect on energy production, mood, muscle function and hormone metabolism. Curiously there are no physical or skin signs of a mild deficiency.

Magnesium is definitely an important piece of the puzzle of PMS.

Iron

It is probably better known that menstruating women have an increased need for the mineral iron; in fact, iron levels are at their lowest four days pre-menstrually. This time there is an RDA (Recommended Daily Allowance) in the UK for iron, which is 12 mg per day; this is somewhat lower than the RDA for the USA, which is 18mg.

The Booker Health Report showed that 60 per cent of females between the ages of 18 and 54 have iron levels below the recommended daily allowance. In another study in 1984, it was found that a group of 15–25-year-old women consumed only 75 per cent of the RDA for iron, so many are at risk of deficiency.

Consuming a cup of tea with a meal will reduce the absorption of iron from all non-animal foods in the diet and from iron supplements.

Zinc and other trace minerals

Zinc, like iron, is an essential mineral which is required in tiny amounts but also plays an important part in many aspects of the body's normal functioning. It is needed for normal hormone production, certain aspects of brain chemistry, for healthy skin and good resistance to infection. The average daily intake of this mineral for women of child-bearing age in the UK is 7.6 mg per day, which compares favourably with an average recommended daily intake of 5.5 mg. However, like iron and magnesium, a significant percentage, at least five, consume less than the recommended minimum of 4.0 mg per day. Furthermore, the absorption of this mineral is easily upset by alcohol, tea, probably coffee, bran, unleavened breads, chapattis, and many other foods. So a considerable percentage of women may be getting insufficient zinc. Any ill-effects are likely to be slight and subtle, but a deficiency certainly could be a contributing factor to some PMS symptoms.

We are not certain about other trace nutrients. If you are eating a healthy diet with plenty of fruit and vegetables and not smoking or drinking then you are likely to have a good intake of the trace nutrients such as selenium, chromium, copper and manganese. A lack of chromium or selenium may occasionally be relevant for some women with PMS. For example, a lack of chromium does have an influence on the action of insulin and the control of blood sugar. Chromium can enhance the effect of insulin, and correcting a deficiency has been shown to improve blood sugar control. This can be important for some women who are either very overweight or eat a diet very high in sugar and refined foods which are depleted of chromium.

IT'S A POOR SHOW

It seems astonishing to consider that such important nutrients are acknowledged to be in such short supply, and yet not a great deal is being done to reverse the trend. Three out of four of these nutrients do not even have a Recommended Daily Allowance in the UK.

When you read the section on Vitamins and Minerals in Chapter 14, pay particular attention to these four important nutrients, notice what their function is in the body and what happens to us if we don't get them in sufficient quantities. Is it any wonder that our bodies are slowly going to seed when we are not providing them with the essential materials they need in order for them to function properly?

In the Self-Help section, I concentrate on foods that contain a high level of these particular nutrients as well as a few others. I will help you to work out a diet for yourself which will provide you with good amounts of the essential nutrients that you are most likely to be short of.

Other barriers

Not only may we be taking in insufficient amounts of vitamins and minerals, but the value of many of these nutrients is impaired by factors like alcohol, tea, coffee and tobacco.

Another thing to bear in mind which severely lowers the nutritional value of food is the cooking process. For example, boiling a cabbage rids it of about 75 per cent of its vitamin C. Baking or frying food can destroy up to 50 per cent of other vitamins. Commercially frozen vegetables can also be lacking in some nutrients by as much as 47 per cent though usually they are the next best thing to fresh ones, since canning can result in up to 70 per cent of the nutritional content being lost. It appears that processing food does little to enhance our health at the end of the day.

A good example of the effect of processing on nutrient content, is the nutrient content of some of McDonald's foods. I am sorry to keep using them as an example, but at least they are one of the few fast-food manufacturers who have had the nerve to assess the nutrient content of their own products.

By now you no doubt realize that a 'normal healthy diet' is somewhat of a myth. Although it is possible to eat a nutritious diet, you need to be fairly educated on the subject before you can even make a start. Then, as you can see, there are numerous hurdles to be overcome.

Whilst all these facts do seem depressing, there is a light at the end of the tunnel. In the Self-Help section on diet I will be concentrating on which types of foods to buy, and suggesting methods of preparation that will preserve the nutrients in your food.

TIMES DO CHANGE

Is it any wonder women suffer with PMS! One hundred years ago, meat, animal fat and sugar were a much smaller part of our diets than today. The consumption of cereal fibres has also dropped by as much as 90 per cent.

These are important factors in relation to PMS, as you will see.

It has become far more difficult to eat a 'normal healthy diet'. However, if you concentrate on avoiding the nutrient-deficient and contaminated foods listed below, you will be making changes for the better in your diet, which will not only help your PMS, but will help you feel healthier all round. There is less you can do to combat the unhealthy effects of the polluted environment, but I make some suggestions below.

The diet of our ancestors. When we examine the diet of our ancestors, we then begin to realize that it is not 'natural' to eat meat in the quantity that the majority of us do today. Evidence shows that diet approximately three million years ago consisted largely of hard seeds, plant fibre, some roots and stems – a diet high in vegetable matter similar to that of the Guinea baboon today.

Animals today are bred to be fat. Modern meat contains some seven times more fat than the wild meat our ancestors ate. Our ancestors' meat also contained five times more of the good polyunsaturated fats than today's meat, which is high in the potentially harmful saturated fats. The ancient diet was also richer in vitamins and minerals and polyunsaturated fats, and many times richer than the modern diet. It was a diet which was largely composed of fresh raw foods.

Even as recently as 50 years ago we were consuming four proper meals per day with one between-meal snack. By the mid-1990s the tables had turned and found us consuming one or two meals per day, not necessarily freshly shopped for or home cooked, and a staggering four between-meal snacks. Our bodies were not designed to be treated in this way.

Antibiotics. Because antibiotics are being so widely used on animals, the conditions that would normally be treated by antibiotics are becoming resistant to them. Apart from being used as a medicine for individual sick animals, they are given to whole herds as a preventive measure, and they are again used for growth promotion.

My advice is to try to use organic or additive-free meat where possible, meat which has not been subjected to drugs, growth promoters or contaminated foods. It's probably better to avoid beef at this time because of mad cow disease. At least PMS is curable! Organic and additive-free meat is becoming more and more available. Certainly local farms and even supermarkets often keep stocks. If you can find 'clean' meat, it can be included in your diet approximately three times per week. An alternative is to limit one's meat intake to moderate quantities of good-quality lean meat, or to become a vegetarian. It's the fat in the meat that will carry much of the pollutants, so avoid it – and also rely more on fish. When eating chicken, don't eat the skin and don't make the gravy from the fatty part of the juices, pour it off first.

Fat consumption. Britain has the honour of having the highest incidence of heart disease in the world. This was not so in the past, when other countries such as Finland and Australia were way ahead. Something drastic must have happened to change statistics so dramatically.

It seems that the saturated fats increase the level of cholesterol which leaves the bloodstream and settles down in the arteries, resulting in a gradual blockage of those supplying the heart, brain and other organs. This leads to heart attacks, strokes and poor circulation. Smoking accelerates the process.

By 1966 the Australian and US rate of heart disease began to decline, but that was not so for Britain, whose casualties were on the increase.

In other countries such as Finland, for example, who were previously 'top of the coronary pops', a national nutritional education campaign was undertaken. The result now is that they are a much healthier nation with a far lower incidence of heart disease than many other countries.

The sweet facts. Over the past 100 years there has been a 25-fold increase in world sugar production. This is a real change from the days when sugar was an expensive luxury that we locked away for high days and holidays, and was only consumed by the wealthy. Refined sugars simply didn't exist for our ancestors. Their diet consisted mainly of vegetables, fruit, cereals and some wild meat. It wasn't until this century that we developed an addiction to the sweet and sticky sugar family.

We clearly don't need refined sugar. What seems to have been overlooked is that our bodies can change complex carbohydrates and proteins into the sugar they require. Sugar contains no vitamins, no minerals, no protein, no fibre, no starches. It may contain tiny traces of calcium and magnesium if you're lucky, and it certainly provides us with loads of calories (kjs), 'empty calories'.

It is actually a fair skill these days not to consume large amounts of sugar, because it is added to so many foods. What do you think the following have in common? Cheese, biscuits, fruit yogurt, tomato sauce, baked beans, pickled cucumbers, muesli, beefburgers, Worcester sauce, pork sausages, peas, cornflakes and Coca-Cola – well, they can all contain sugar. Coca-Cola contains some eight teaspoonfuls per can.

There are some more nutritious alternatives which I will discuss in the Self-Help section. The food manufacturers are beginning to understand that their consumers are waking up, and the majority actually don't want to be dumped on. For now my advice is to read the labels carefully when you are shopping: I guarantee you will have a few surprises!

Water

Our most important nutrient is water, and sadly it is becoming one of our major sources of pollution. Not only is the water contaminated with lead, aluminium and copper, we now have nitrates to contend with as well. Nitrates are chemicals used in fertilizers to promote crop growth.

Why are nitrates harmful? Well, they go through chemical changes and at the end of the day turn into nitrosamines which are believed to be strong cancer-producing chemicals.

Toxic minerals

Toxic minerals in the form of lead and mercury are in the soil, the air and the water, as well as being present in our food. During this century their levels have been rising rapidly, and at times to a point where our bodies have not been able to cope.

Lead. Lead pollution has been much discussed in the media over the past few years. High lead levels are acknowledged to be linked to low birth weight and low intelligence in children. As a result of extensive research on lead, many countries have removed lead from petrol and are trying to keep lead levels down in cities. However, it is far more difficult to remove it from the water supply as the filtering systems at water purification plants can't always cope with the load.

Helpful tips to avoid the toxins

- Concentrate on eating a nutritious diet, particularly high in zinc, magnesium, calcium and vitamins C and B.

- Take a well-balanced multi-vitamin supplement and some extra vitamin C if you are at particular risk.

- Scrub all fruit and vegetables with a brush to clean off as many toxins as possible, and remove the outer layers of lettuce and cabbage, etc. Don't peel fruit and vegetables unless you don't like the peel – very often the bulk of the nutrients is just under the skin. Use organic vegetables and salad stuff or grow your own where possible, without using chemicals.

- Water filters tend to filter out a good deal of the toxic metals. Water purifiers can be bought in healthfood shops, but they aren't so efficient. Every so often the filter needs replacing – and it's amazing what collects in it. Rather the toxic deposits collect in the filter than your body!

Avoid:

- Spending too much time near busy roads if the local exhaust fumes contain lead (which may be easier said than done).

- Copper and aluminium cookware unless with a non-stick lining.

- Alcohol, as it increases lead absorption.

- Refined foods which give the body little protection against toxins.

- Antacids which contain aluminium salts.

Food additives

Whilst, of course, there are some perfectly harmless substances added to food, the number of potentially harmful additives is significant. Many additives have been shown to cause hyperactivity in children, asthma, eczema, skin rashes and swelling. It's obviously important to be able to differentiate between the safe and not-so-safe additives.

After being bombarded by warnings about additives is it any wonder that some of us have at one time or another avoided all foods containing them? Understandably, 'additive' has become a dirty word in some circles. But it's important to understand that some additives are, in fact, beneficial! For example: beneficial additives include riboflavin – vitamin B2 – and calcium L-Ascorbate which is vitamin C, and the many preservatives which help keep our food from spoiling.

WHICH ADDITIVES ARE SAFE?

Fortunately, there is now no need to remain confused about which additives are safe and which are potentially harmful. Look in Appendix 2 on page 272 for details of booklets and books on additives which will help you to pick out the dangerous additives from the safe ones.

Coffee

Over the last 10 years reports have begun to filter through about the health hazards attached to coffee consumption. Probably one of the reasons why these facts are now coming to light is that increasing amounts of coffee are being consumed. Since 1950 the consumption of coffee in the UK has increased fourfold and according to the US Department of Agriculture, in 1994 21.1 gallons (80 litres) of coffee were consumed per person per annum in the USA. Many people become quite addicted to it unknowingly, and couldn't give up the habit easily.

We now know that coffee worsens nervous tension, anxiety and insomnia. So obviously, no matter how much we may enjoy it, drinking coffee to excess is not a healthy habit. In fact, coffee contains caffeine which is a mental and physical stimulant. This can be of benefit of course, but even with 2–4 cups per day, adverse effects can be experienced. These include anxiety, restlessness, nervousness, insomnia, rapid pulse, palpitations, shakes and passing increased quantities of water. Regular coffee drinkers not only enjoy the flavour, but in many cases come to rely on the stimulation to get them through the day. If you cannot get going without your first fix of the day, you know what I mean!

Weaning yourself off coffee can sometimes be a fairly traumatic experience. It can sometimes produce symptoms not unlike a drug withdrawal, in particular a severe headache, which may take several days to disappear. However, rest assured they do eventually go completely, as long as you manage to abstain from coffee.

Ways to go about giving up coffee

- Cut down gradually over the space of a week or two.

- Use decaffeinated coffee instead of coffee containing caffeine, but limit yourself to 2–3 cups per day. However if you suffer from premenstrual breast problems it is better to avoid it altogether as the chemical called methylxanthines can aggravate breast problems.

- Try alternative drinks like Barleycup or Bambu which you can obtain from healthfood shops.

- If you like filter coffee, you can still use your filter, but with decaffeinated versions or with roasted dandelion root instead of coffee. You can obtain dried roasted dandelion root from good healthfood shops. It may sound a bit way out, but it has a very pleasant malted flavour.

Tea

The British are famous for their tea consumption. Tea, like coffee, contains caffeine, about 50 mg per cup, compared to coffee's 100 mg per strong cup. Tea also contains tannin, which inhibits the absorption of zinc and iron in particular. Excess tea produces the same effects as coffee, and you can also experience a withdrawal headache. Tea can also cause constipation.

By drinking a cup of tea with a meal you can cut down the absorption of iron from vegetarian foods to one-third. Whereas, a glass of fresh orange juice with the same meal would increase iron absorption by two times because of its high vitamin C content. Vegetarian and vegan women need their intake of iron to be readily absorbed. Therefore, drinking anything other than small amounts of weak tea may mean they risk becoming iron deficient.

'Herbal teas' don't count as tea as such. It's really a confusing name. Most herbal teas are free of caffeine and tannin and just consist of a collection of herbs. Unlike regular tea, they can be cleansing and relaxing.

Alcohol

Alcohol is causing far greater problems to our society than most of us realize. It is the drug most seriously abused. Young people tend to begin drinking at an earlier age than was the case in previous generations. Public attitudes to drinking have become much more liberal and gradually alcohol has become widely socially accepted, without an appreciation of its adverse effects.

A major factor explaining the rise in alcohol consumption appears to be the decline in the real price of alcohol. It's not alcohol itself that has gone down in price, but the amount of work necessary to earn the cost of a drink.

Before I go any further I must state that I am not addressing alcoholics as such in this section but 'social drinkers'; those who like to have a few drinks, two or three times a week, can be jeopardizing their health. Anything above the national average for women, that is one glass of wine or half a pint of beer or one sherry or vermouth per day, means running some degree of health risk. Men consume on average three times this amount, and are recommended to halve it.

Alcohol in excess destroys body tissue over the years, and can cause or contribute to many diseases. For example, cardiovascular diseases, digestive disorders, inflammation and ulceration of the lining of the digestive tract, liver disease, brain degeneration, miscarriages, damage to unborn children and malnutrition, are some of the conditions associated with the long-term use of alcohol. In particular, certain vitamins and minerals are destroyed or lost from the body, including vitamin B1, thiamin, magnesium, zinc, vitamin B6, pyridoxine, calcium and vitamin D. All of these nutrients are particularly important to PMS sufferers, as you will see in Chapter 14.

As most of these conditions come on gradually, we often don't see the real dangers of alcohol. There is no impact like that of an accident, or the drama of an ambulance arriving to carry you off. But instead, there is a slow process of destruction which conveniently escapes our awareness.

Amongst those PMS sufferers who like a regular drink are those who increase their consumption considerably before their period. If this happens to you, then you will be well aware of the social problems that go with it, such as mood swings and personality changes. When this occurs others around become affected, and relationships may be strained at home and at work. It is a fact that one-third of the divorce petitions cite alcohol as a contributory factor and one-third of child abuse cases are linked to heavy drinking by a parent. Local courtrooms are always having to deal with people who committed offences whilst under the influence of alcohol. Offences that might never have been committed, were it not for that 'one for the road'!

Old habits die hard

The type of food you eat is usually determined by you. However, there are many other factors that influence your 'preferences' through your life. The two main influential factors are:

1   Your parents, who introduce you to your initial diet, based on their preferences and their knowledge about diet.

The chances are that you continue to eat many of the foods introduced to you by your parents through your life. Habit patterns are quite hard to change, and a very important factor, of course, is that you've got to want to change them.

2   The exposure to the media which we all have in the form of advertisements on television, in magazines, billboards, etc. Now, the second factor, the power of persuasion via the media, might be highly desirable – if it was good food that was being promoted. If the media were dedicated to educating the public about a good, wholesome, nutritious diet, a more valuable asset we could not wish for! In reality they are there to persuade

us, on behalf of the food industry, that fast foods, processed foods, or convenience foods, call them what you will, are desirable. They would have us believe that coffee is sexy and that we should switch to cola-based drinks for energy.

Rather than being a help educationally, they are often a great hindrance. Considering how much television we watch, is it any wonder that the hypnotic powers of the media begin to affect many of us, who would otherwise be influenced by common sense and our own good judgement?

Take one positive step at a time

I am sorry to bombard you with so many depressing facts all at once. We the consumers definitely need more information about the food we eat and the environmental factors we are subjected to.

Probably the first step towards reversing the effects of the twentieth century on your body is for you to acknowledge the value of that body if you haven't already done so. After all, we only have one body to last us through a lifetime, so it's important to treat it with respect.

It's up to you how often you expose your body to alcohol, cigarettes, drugs and additives, and how physically fit you keep through exercise. Making one change at a time is better than not changing at all. I will be concentrating on how to go about making changes in the Self-Help section of the book, Part Three.

As for environmental pollution, there are now many worthwhile national and local groups running campaigns to help overcome these problems. You will find a list of these in Part Four. If you are concerned about your local situation, you can always contact the government representative for your area for help and advice.

If you have been neglecting your body to some extent, now may be the time to take stock. Don't expect your doctor to piece you back together again when you have fallen apart through 'environmental wear and nutritional tear'!

It's up to each one of us to look after our bodies to the best of our abilities and to treat them as well as any other of our treasured possessions.

12

MEDICAL TREATMENTS

There are now many different treatments for PMS. The last 12 years in particular have seen a flourish of medical publications reporting the effects of a wide variety of different treatment approaches. Their conflicting findings can create more confusion than clarification for both the sufferer and the doctor.

It is understandably hard to imagine why so many different treatments, both hormonal and non-hormonal, can all appear to be effective in treating one condition. Much of the confusion arises because many of the studies conducted have involved only small numbers of women, and have only been performed once, which is really insufficient to prove anything. Also, some of the studies haven't assessed PMS symptoms thoroughly, or explored the possible side-effects of treatment in detail. As a result, we are still in the dark about how effective many of these preparations are in the treatment of PMS.

That said, if we are careful in interpreting these trials, then they can usefully increase our understanding of PMS, and improve the care we can offer to sufferers, especially those with symptoms which may have proved difficult to treat. In an attempt to put the technical findings in perspective, the rest of this chapter is therefore a brief review of the different hormonal and non-hormonal treatments that have ever been tried in PMS. For the technically minded, the relevant references given in the appendix of the book are on page 285.

HORMONAL TREATMENTS FOR PMS

Many of the hormonal treatments that have been put forward as treatments for PMS have been based on the notion that PMS was due to a lack of a particular hormone. Research of the last 15 years has, as we have already seen, laid that idea firmly to rest. Even so, some of the more powerful hormonal preparations have been shown to be effective. How could this be? The production of true pre-menstrual symptoms is undoubtedly linked to the normal hormonal cycle. Any treatment that abolishes or suppresses normal hormone production by the ovaries will alter premenstrual symptoms for the better, especially if the symptoms are severe to start with. The difficulty with using these types of treatments is that they can produce considerable side-effects, both in the short and long term.

Coming off hormonal preparations may not be easy as they rarely correct the underlying reasons for pre-menstrual symptoms, and the symptoms are likely to return with a vengeance when you stop taking them. Additionally, they are often very expensive. On balance, there seems little justification for using many hormonal products, though we appreciate they may occasionally be useful for individual patients.

PROGESTERONE PREPARATIONS

Progesterone is one of the two main hormones produced by the ovaries. It was once believed that deficiency of this hormone was the cause of PMS, but this is now known not to be the case.

Progesterone pessaries (Cyclogest)

Progesterone, in the form of a pessary inserted into the vagina, has been one of the most popular treatments for PMS. However, eight different scientific studies showed very little evidence of any benefit. The largest of these studies by Dr Freeman and colleagues from the University of Pennsylvania involved 168 women. Those who were given progesterone showed no benefit when compared with women who took a placebo (inactive agent). The progesterone which is normally given for 10 to 14 days before the onset of menstruation can no longer be considered as an effective treatment for PMS.

The latest trial on progesterone involved British women, and contrary to all its predecessors, showed a very small benefit in those who took progesterone compared with those who took a placebo. Interpretation of this trial must be cautious as the number of women who dropped out during the study was particularly high and the degree of benefit was minimal.

Overall, one can conclude that progesterone pessaries may be helpful for a few women but cannot be regarded as a routinely effective treatment.

Progesterone tablets

The natural hormone, progesterone, is not active by mouth. Thus for oral preparations synthetic progesterones, known as progestagens, need to be given. Dydrogesterone is one such synthetic progestagen that has been tried in PMS. It has shown modest success in two out of four trials, when compared with placebos. It may also be effective for painful periods and endometriosis, and is particularly suited for women who have PMS and one or both of these conditions together.

Norethisterone is another synthetic progesterone used in the treatment of PMS, though it has not been subjected to much scientific scrutiny. It is effective in the treatment of heavy periods, or delays periods that occur too frequently, and is again best reserved for women who have these problems in addition to PMS.

THE ORAL CONTRACEPTIVE PILL

There are many different types of Pill. Since they were first used in the 1960s, the dosage of oestrogen and progesterone that they contain has fallen dramatically, and with it the risk of side-effects.

The Pill has a variable effect on PMS. In some women it may make it worse, and in others it may improve it; in many it makes little or no difference. It cannot be considered a routine treatment for PMS, but it may be worth trying in women with mild to moderate PMS who require this type of contraception. One type of combined oral contraceptive pill containing ethinyloestradiol and norgstimate (Cilest) has been shown to be mildly effective in helping pre-menstrual symptomatology and for some this may be the first choice of pill for those with PMS. It should be noted that the Pill can aggravate migraine headaches, and cause an increase in blood pressure in some sensitive women. Women who are overweight, smoke or who have high blood pressure probably should not consider the Pill as an option anyway.

OESTROGEN PREPARATIONS AND HORMONE REPLACEMENT THERAPY (HRT)

Oestrogen can come in forms other than the oral contraceptive pill and some of these have been tried in PMS.

Oestrogen implants which are inserted under the skin of the abdomen by a small operation under local anaesthetic have been popularized by Mr John Studd from King's College Hospital, London. He and his colleagues have found them to be highly effective in the treatment of PMS, but they cannot be used long-term because of side-effects, and because the body adapts to the artificially high levels of oestrogen. We have seen a number of women who have had considerable problems with this method of treating their PMS. Despite high, sometimes excessively high, levels of circulating oestrogen they experienced breakthrough symptoms as well as sometimes hot flushes and night sweats. In such a situation a mixture of physical and mental symptoms may persist until oestrogen levels fall back into the normal range, which may take up to a year. It is now considered good practice that those women who require oestrogen implants have a blood test before each implant to ensure that oestrogen levels do not rise excessively.

Oestrogen given in the form of a patch which slowly releases the hormone into the bloodstream is an elegant and more gentle way of administering this hormone. This may also be an effective treatment for PMS, but is best reserved for women who are approaching the menopause.

When taking oestrogen, you will also need to take progesterone in order to maintain your monthly bleed, unless you have had a hysterectomy.

TESTOSTERONE – THE MALE HORMONE

It may surprise you to know that this hormone, in the form of an implant, has been tried in the treatment of PMS, with some benefit for depressive symptoms but not for physical complaints. It is not a routine treatment.

OTHER HORMONE-RELATED PREPARATIONS

There are a number of other powerful drugs which influence hormone metabolism that have been used in PMS. They can often produce side-effects and are best reserved for special situations.

Danazol:

This drug blocks or interferes with the action of many sex hormones. It can be useful in situations where there is a hormone excess, but anything other than small doses can lead to side-effects, including excessive hair growth, deepening of the voice and other changes. Low doses can be effective in PMS, and are also useful in the treatment of endometriosis, heavy periods and pre-menstrual breast tenderness, if all else fails.

Bromocriptine:

This is another powerful drug which blocks the effect of the hormone, pro-lactin, from the pituitary gland. It too can be used for pre-menstrual breast tenderness, and in small doses to help PMS, but again it is not suitable for long-term treatment of PMS.

Others

Certain drugs can treat PMS very successfully, by switching off the pituitary gland's stimulus to the ovaries. In this way the ovaries go into 'retirement' and a false menopause is achieved. This abolishes the pre-menstrual symptoms, but not surprisingly replaces them with hot flushes and the risk of osteoporosis. This is really a last-ditch treatment, and has no place for the majority of sufferers.

DRUG TREATMENTS FOR PMS

Just as almost every kind of hormonal treatment has been used in the treatment of PMS, so has almost every type of drug been tried. Many of these treatments have not established themselves as routine therapies.

Anti-depressants

Historically, anti-depressants have not been used much in the treatment of PMS until recently. Despite depression being a common feature of PMS anti-depressants rarely work in women whose depression was purely cyclical.

In recent years there have been several trials of the popular anti-depressant Fluoxetine, commonly known as Prozac. This drug is used mainly in the treatment of depression and the eating disorder bulimia nervosa where craving and bingeing on foods is a central feature. It can also be effective in PMS in about 60 per cent of cases according to American studies. It works by altering the level of mood-altering chemi-cals in the brain, in particular that of serotonin. The very fact that this anti-depressant can actually work requires us to combine theories about hormonal chemistry with those of nervous system chemistry in the causa-tion of PMS.

For many women the problem with taking this type of drug is that they may experience side-effects including nausea, vomiting, increased anxiety and panic attacks, insomnia, drowsiness and aches and pains. In this respect it may make some women's pre-menstrual symptoms worse, especially those already suffering with panic attacks and anxiety. More importantly, however, many women do not wish to take this sort of preparation for fear of psychological dependency on a mood-altering drug. That said, it is useful to have a potent anti-depressant that helps PMS. For those with severe depression who are at risk of suicide this sort of drug may represent a useful addition to their treatment.

Diuretics (water tablets)

This in the past has been a popular treatment, particularly in the treatment of pre-menstrual fluid retention and breast tenderness. Many older types of diuretics are effective in the short term, but lead to a loss of the important minerals, magnesium and potassium. Magnesium may be low in some 50 per cent of women with PMS, so further losses would not be desirable. Diuretics are not expected to help mood changes. One type of diuretic, called Spironolactone, has been shown to be moderately helpful, but its manufacturer no longer recommends it for long-term use in young patients.

Most of the symptoms of fluid retention should respond to a diet that is low in sodium (salt) and, if necessary, restricted in calories.

Pain-killers

These can be useful for painful periods, migraine and other headaches that occur just before or with the period. One type of pain-killer, available on prescription only, is Mefenamic acid, which when taken for two weeks before the onset of menstruation may help PMS symptoms. If you experience very painful periods you should ask your doctor for a gynaecological assessment.

Sleeping tablets, sedatives and anti-anxiety drugs

The over-use of these drugs by the medical profession has been of particular concern to many patients over the last 30 years. They have no role in the treatment of PMS, except perhaps occasionally for short-term use in the treatment of anxiety or insomnia. One type of anti-anxiety drug, Buspirone, has shown some benefit in one small trial in PMS. The method of assessing its benefit was, however, limited.

All of these types of drugs should be used with great caution, if at all, and patients should always be given advice about other measures to limit or control anxiety.

Antibiotics

Extraordinary as it may seem, there has even been a trial of antibiotics in PMS! This involved giving an old, established antibiotic, Doxycycline, to a group of women aged 25 to 35 years, 77 per cent of whom also had evidence of vaginal infection. The reduction in PMS symptoms was accompanied by a clearance of the associated vaginal infection. Other doctors have related PMS to vaginal infection with *Candida albicans*, a yeast that causes thrush. The message here is simple. If there is evidence of vaginal or other infection, then treat it. In doing so one may help PMS as well.

Other treatments

Many other treatments have been reported as being tried in PMS, including lithium (a drug used to treat certain mental illnesses). Three studies showed no benefit; Naltrexone (a drug used to counteract the side-effects of morphine) showed benefit in one small study when given at mid-cycle; and an anti-allergy treatment showed benefit in one study, especially in those with an allergic tendency.

Let me finish this chapter with a few conclusions which I hope will help you make sense of the situation.
1. Do not accept a treatment as proven to be effective unless it has shown benefit in at least two studies.
2. Powerful hormone and drug treatments probably are effective, but at the cost of significant short- or long-term side-effects. They are best reserved as a last resort.
3. All treatments can, and should ideally always, be combined with self-help and nutritional treatments.
4. Many of the above treatments are best suited to those women who have PMS with associated problems, including period pains, vaginal infection, gynaecological problems, or who are approaching menopause.
5. Many experts now agree that a nutritional approach to PMS is indeed the best first-line treatment. As the nutritional approach is so effective, there will usually be no need to make use of hormonal and drug treatments.

13

NUTRITIONAL TREATMENTS

Thankfully, in the last few years nutritional treatments for PMS have been taken more seriously. This has come about because of the wider apprecia- tion that many existing medical treatments are not as effective as was once thought and often produce undesirable side-effects, whereas research has shown the value of some nutritional preparations which, as a rule, have no side-effects.

A wide variety of nutritional products have been assessed for PMS, including individual vitamins and minerals, combinations of vitamins and minerals, and evening primrose oil, which contains some specialized fats with vitamin-like qualities. The reason why most of these nutrients were tried in the first place was because of the way in which they are known to influence the function of either hormones or the chemistry of the brain and nervous system, and thus, potentially, the body's metabolism, for the better. But how effective are they?

VITAMIN B6 (PYRIDOXINE)

This has been the most popular nutritional preparation for PMS in years past. Studies conducted in the UK, the Netherlands and Australia have, surprisingly, not found that deficiency of this vitamin is a particular feature of women with PMS, though mild deficiency is quite common in people experiencing anxiety, depression and other mental symptoms. However, it is now known that vitamin B6 influences the action of the hormone oestrogen in the body, as well as being important in the normal function of the nervous system and the processing of protein-rich foods.

Vitamin B6 was the subject of a health warning from the Department of Health in December 1996. Some advisors to the Government were concerned that excessive amounts of Vitamin B6 could cause damage to the nervous system. Close examination of this issue has confirmed that this can occur at doses of at least 500 mg per day or more. The Department of Health took an extremely cautious and unfounded view that the public should consume no more than 10mg per day. We and many other experts felt that this advice was incorrect as we had never seen a problem at up to 300 mg per day and to our knowledge no confirmed reports of Vitamin B6 induced nerve damage have occurred in the UK or with the use of Optivite worldwide. It is likely that the effective dose of Vitamin B6 for PMS is at least 50 mg and restricting the daily dose to 10 mg would deprive many women of potentially helpful treatment. Consequently we have not changed our policy but continue to recommend doses of Vitamin B6 up to 300 mg per day combined with magnesium and other vitamins in patients who are supervised by ourselves, their doctor or other experienced practitioner. For the general public an appropriate recommendation would be not to exceed 200 mg of vitamin B6 per day, preferably taken in conjunction with other B vitamins and the mineral magnesium.

VITAMIN E

This has long been a popular supplement since it was shown to prevent miscarriages in pregnant rats! Actual deficiency in humans is exceptionally rare, but vitamin E can influence the body's metabolism of fats, which in turn can influence hormone and nervous system chemistry.

Three studies of vitamin E have been performed, all of which have been conducted in the United States. Two of the three studies showed benefit with, curiously, the most effective dosage being 300 to 400 IU (International Units) per day, rather than a higher dose. This may be because different dosages have different effects on female hormones. Certainly it is worth considering; it may help depressive symptoms the most.

MAGNESIUM

Magnesium has, until recently, been a neglected nutrient. For much of this century it has only been considered worthy for use as a laxative. However, it is known to be essential for muscle, nerve and bone function and structure.

The typical diet of developed civilizations can be low in this nutrient if there is over-reliance on convenience foods; an excellent dietary source is green vegetables.

It had been suggested by French workers in the 1970s that a mild lack of magnesium might contribute to anxiety and related symptoms. Dr Guy Abraham, from the United States, together with his colleague, Dr Lubran, were the first to show that many, but not all, women with PMS have evidence of a mild deficit of this mineral – a reduced concentration was found in the red blood cells of sufferers when compared with healthy women. This finding has been confirmed in a number of studies including two of our own, and now is perhaps the most consistent abnormal finding in women with PMS.

In addition to PMS, magnesium has been studied in a number of common related conditions. Many of these studies show either that poor intake is associated with a particular health problem or that supplements may produce mild benefit. Such conditions include constipation, muscle aches and pains (fibromyalgia), muscle cramps, high blood pressure, migraine headaches and fatigue. Even a tendency to wheeze has been associated with poor dietary intakes of magnesium. Many of the beneficial effects of magnesium are attributable to its effects on muscles where it aids their relaxation. Diets high in salt which are very common, disturb the balance of this important mineral. Thus PMS sufferers with some of the above complaints may particularly benefit from this useful mineral.

Unfortunately, only one trial of magnesium alone has been undertaken, and this was by a group of Italian doctors who administered 375 mg per day of this nutrient for two months. There was a significant rise in the level of magnesium and an accompanying fall in the level of pre-menstrual symptoms reported. This important study deserves repetition. Certainly, magnesium is a very promising preparation. It is particularly useful for constipation – it is interesting to note that severe constipation in young women is associated with quite marked hormonal abnormalities.

Magnesium comes in different forms, the most convenient being a tablet. Liquid preparations and crystals of magnesium sulphate (Epsom Salts) are only really useful as laxatives.

MULTI-VITAMINS

Rather than buy them individually, it would seem tempting to use nutritional supplements that combine several nutrients in one preparation. This idea has its merits. It is known that many individual nutrients interact, requiring the presence of their fellows to function properly, and that when someone is deficient in one nutrient, they are likely to be lacking in others as well.

A number of multi-vitamins, usually with minerals, have found their way on to the marketplace in different countries around the world. Virtually all of these preparations have been used without being assessed scientifically. The only preparation of this type that has been subjected to trials published in proper medical journals is Optivite. This preparation is a comprehensive multi-vitamin and mineral supplement that contains substantial amounts of vitamin B6, other vitamins, magnesium and other minerals. It has been the subject of several open or preliminary trials and, more importantly, it has been assessed in four scientific trials where it has been compared with placebo or 'dummy' tablets. The conclusion of these trials from both the United Kingdom and the United States is that it is an effective treatment for PMS when given over three menstrual cycles. The most effective dosage is six tablets a day, every day throughout the menstrual cycle. The effectiveness of this particular supplement may be enhanced by combining it with dietary modification and also exercise. This has very much been our experience at the WNAS in our many years of using this and other nutritional preparations. Interestingly, there is evidence from one American study that Optivite, when combined with dietary changes, does produce a potentially beneficial effect on the metabolism of female sex hormones.

EVENING PRIMROSE OIL

In the 1980s, evening primrose oil became an increasingly popular supplement, and has been the subject of many trials in PMS and other conditions. The particular attraction of EPO is that this oil is rich in an essential fat called gamma-linolenic acid, low levels of which have been recorded in some women with PMS. This interesting fat, and its chemical relatives, does have some influence on hormone metabolism and many aspects of body health. It seems that some individuals may lack the ability to make sufficient amounts of gamma-linolenic acid from other fats in the diet, such as those provided by sunflower and other vegetable oils.

The evidence from scientific trials shows that EPO may be of particular benefit for pre-menstrual breast tenderness, but may not be so helpful for other symptoms. Like Optivite it is best taken when following a healthy diet, as alcohol and a lack of many other nutrients interferes with this delicate area of body metabolism.

The most effective dose of evening primrose oil is 3 to 4 g per day, usually as six to eight 500 mg capsules taken every day through the menstrual cycle. It needs to be taken for four to six cycles, as breast symptoms can be quite stubborn.

The effectiveness of other plant oil preparations, such as blackcurrant seed, starflower oil or borage oil in PMS, is not known as trials have not been conducted. They cannot therefore be recommended.

SIDE-EFFECTS OF NUTRITIONAL PREPARATIONS

No review of the above supplements is complete without mentioning that all of them can produce side-effects, though these are rare and usually much less serious than those that occur with drug-based preparations.

Very high doses of vitamin B6 (pyridoxine) can produce mild nerve damage, causing numbness or tingling in the hands or feet. This has only definitely been described at doses of 500 mg or more per day, as a single nutrient, on a regular basis. Optivite at the effective dosage of six tablets per day provides 300 mg per day of pyridoxine in a slow-release preparation. Nerve damage with this preparation, even at higher doses, has not been reported in any of its numerous trials, nor in the many years of its use, either in the US or the UK.

The main side-effect of magnesium is diarrhoea, which quickly alerts the user to reduce the dose. Magnesium should not be taken by those with poor kidney function, unless under medical supervision, as excessive amounts may accumulate in the body.

Evening primrose oil should not be taken by anyone suffering with epilepsy, as occasionally this condition may be worsened by its use. Again, medical advice should be sought.

All nutritional products may occasionally cause minor symptoms such as nausea, slight abdominal discomfort, diarrhoea or headache. If this occurs they should be stopped for a few days and then tried again at a lower dose. Alternatively, you should obtain some professional advice.

It is unlikely that you will need to take any of these or other nutritional preparations at high or full dosage in the long term. If they prove to be effective, the dose can be reduced, and if not effective, then they should be stopped and a different treatment tried. Some women do find that it is helpful to continue with a modest dose of some supplements, such as vitamin B, Optivite, Femvite (one or two tablets per day) or evening primrose oil (one or two capsules per day) in the longer term. These dosages are safe and reasonable.

We find scientifically based supplements to be a very useful nutritional prop in the short term. Once the symptoms are under control the dosages can be cut back, and very often ex-sufferers can manage with their new diet and exercise alone.

14

NUTRITION
AND THE BODY:
VITAMINS AND MINERALS,
WHAT THEY DO

THE BODY

One thing we have in common is that we all have a body! Our body is nothing more nor less than a highly complicated biochemical machine, the function of which, like any engine, is dependent upon the quality of its food or fuel supply. The body is composed of many different organs and tissues which have important and essential functions and interactions. For example, if you want to move your arm, a tiny electrical message passes from the brain, through the nervous system and down the nerves to the muscles in your arm, which then contract. The degree of stretch or tension in a muscle is relayed, via other nerves, back to the brain, so that the muscle does not over-, or under-stretch in performing the movement that you originally intended.

There are factors that affect the healthy function of nerves, muscles and all other parts of the body. *Firstly, you need to inherit a good and healthy metabolism.* The thousands of chemical processes that take place within each and every cell are mainly determined by the genetic material in the centre of the nucleus of the cell. This genetic material is a master plan or blueprint. It holds the key to which chemical reactions need to take place in order for that cell to function. It determines whether a cell is a muscle cell, nerve cell, skin cell, red blood cell, or any other type of cell. Almost everyone has healthy genes, and thus the possibility for their body to be completely healthy and function efficiently. However, there may be subtle individual variations in metabolism, which determine the strengths and weaknesses of one's physical constitution. This may explain why some people are sensitive to some types of dietary change or nutritional deficiencies, and others are not – why some women may develop Pre-Menstrual Syndrome, and others, despite eating an 'unhealthy' diet, may not.

Secondly, some disease states can lead to the development of PMS.

Finally, and most importantly, there must be a healthy diet, giving an adequate supply of those nutrients necessary for the normal functioning of each individual cell. A lack of any one nutrient leads to changes in the cell's metabolism, which in turn will result in changes in the individual's health.

THE DIET

Many people, when they hear the word diet, think of a weight-reducing or slimming diet. The word diet simply refers to the type of food that a person is eating. Every one of us has a diet of some kind, unless we are starving to death. Certain components of a diet are essential, and many of these terms may be familiar to you. The essential nutrients include proteins, fats, carbohydrates, fibre, water, vitamins, minerals and essential fatty acids. Other factors that are also essential for life include a certain degree of heat and light. First, we should have a brief word about what each of these nutrients does, and why they are essential.

Proteins. These are the building blocks of a body. A protein is in fact a group of smaller building blocks called amino acids, which in turn are composed of individual chemicals. Proteins are found in large quantities in tissue such as muscle, skin and bone. In these tissues protein serves a mainly structural function, contributing to the shape of the body, and its ability to move. Other proteins perform highly specialized functions, such as hormones which influence metabolism, and antibodies which help to fight infection.

We all make our own proteins, mainly in the liver, but to do this, must have a steady supply, from our diet, of amino acids, which are in turn derived from the proteins that we eat. Thus, it is essential for us to eat good-quality proteins, such as fish, eggs, nuts, seeds, wholegrains, peas, beans and lentils and lean additive-free meat. A lack of protein in the diet would lead to loss of muscle function and performance, and to a multitude of changes in the body's metabolism.

Fats. These are providers of energy, and, apart from two essential fats (discussed below), are really not necessary to the body at all. However, every type of protein contains some fat, whether it is an animal or vegetable source of protein. This fat can be burnt by the body to provide energy. The liver and muscle cells in particular can make substantial use of fats in this way. Fats also provide a structural role in forming the walls of each individual cell.

The specialized fat, cholesterol, is used to form the male and female hormones, vitamin D and other important hormones in the body. Our bodies can usually make twice as much cholesterol as we eat. So often a raised level of cholesterol in the blood is caused not by eating too much cholesterol, but a faulty metabolism and a high-fat, high-sugar diet. We certainly do not need to increase our intake of animal fats, as I'm sure you will appreciate after reading the section on fats in Chapter 11, page 106.

Essential fatty acids. These are specialized fats, whose importance is becoming increasingly realized. There are two essential fatty acids, linoleic and linolenic acid. As their names suggest, they are very similar in chemical structure, and both of them are of the polyunsaturated type (i.e. not cholesterol-forming). These perform two main roles. First, they are a structural component of the walls of many cells, and thus contribute to the cellular skeleton of the body. Secondly, these two essential fatty acids can be transformed into a wide variety of different chemical compounds which appear to play a part in hormone function and inflammation. Disturbance in the metabolism of these essential fatty acids has been described in one group of women with PMS. However, this has not been confirmed by a second study. Even so, supplements of evening primrose oil, Efamol, have been shown to be effective in the treatment of pre-menstrual breast tenderness, as well as in the skin condition, eczema. It remains to be seen what role these nutrients play in PMS-causation.

Carbohydrates. Carbohydrates, too, are a source of energy. They can be divided into two categories: simple and complex. Simple ones include glucose, fructose (fruit sugar), sucrose (ordinary or table sugar), and lactose (milk sugar). Glucose and fructose are in fact the simplest sugars, consisting of only one type of sugar each. Sucrose and lactose, on the other hand, contain two different types of sugar joined together, and thus are sometimes known as di-saccharides (two sugars).

Polysaccharides (literally, many sugars), are the 'complex' carbohydrates most usually found in vegetables. These consist of many interlinked sugar sub-units, and in order for them to be used by the body, they must be broken down into simple, single-sugar units by the digestive processes in the gut. Vegetables, wholegrains, nuts and seeds are high in these complex carbohydrates.

The refining of sugar cane and sugar beet to make table sugar, sucrose, results in a loss of some of these complex carbohydrates, and a loss in the vitamins, minerals and fibre present in the original plant. When we eat these carbohydrates they are converted by the digestive processes and the body's metabolism to the simple sugar, glucose, which is a major form of energy in the body. Glucose is essential for the brain, as it can only use this form of fuel. However, one does not have to eat glucose or sucrose, table sugar, in order for the brain and nervous system to have an adequate supply: the liver can make glucose from fats or proteins, as well as from other types of sugars, so while glucose is essential for life, it is a mistake to believe we have to add it to the diet. However, some form of carbohydrate, preferably the complex or unrefined carbohydrates, are necessary for an adequate supply of energy.

Fibre. Fibre is the undigestible carbohydrate residues found in food. Natural or unprocessed foods are usually high in fibre and include whole-grains, nuts, seeds and fruit. Some types of carbohydrate cannot be digested by the human body, and so pass through the stomach and digestive tract to the large bowel. Here, fibre absorbs water and other waste materials, and forms our waste product, faeces. A lack of fibre in the diet often leads to constipation, but it is now realized that fibre has other important functions. Lack of fibre is also associated with such conditions as gallstones, varicose veins, obesity, heart disease and diabetes. Of particular relevance is the fact that fibre binds with cholesterol and hormones that are secreted by the liver into the gut. A high-fibre diet may help in expulsion of excessive quantities of cholesterol and unwanted female sex hormones, but more of this later.

Water. This is of course essential for health. Our bodies are composed of 60–70 per cent water, and many bodily functions are dependent upon water. Water is necessary for vitamins, minerals and other chemicals to dissolve in. The amount of urine produced by the kidneys is largely dependent upon the amount of water consumed. An adequate water intake is necessary to clear waste materials through the kidneys, and to allow normal metabolic processes to take place. Water can sometimes be retained by the body, particularly if the intake of salt (sodium) is high. Both salt and water need to be cleared by the kidneys, and their ability to do this may vary from individual to individual. Women who have suffered with pre-menstrual water retention for years, have managed to overcome the condition by making changes to their diet and taking additional supplements.

VITAMINS

Vitamins are the best-known essential nutrient. Indeed, their name was derived from the term 'vital amines' (a type of chemical). They are named as letters of the alphabet, A, B, C, D, E, and K, and members of the B group are further subdivided by numbers into vitamins B1, 2, 3, 5, 6, 12 and Folic acid. The vitamins themselves, as a whole, are divided into two groups. The water-soluble vitamins include members of the vitamin B complex and vitamin C, and the fat-soluble group includes vitamins A, D, E and K.

Vitamins are vital but only in tiny or trace amounts, unlike proteins, carbohydrates and fats, which are necessary in substantial quantities. These trace amounts of vitamins help modify and control essential cellular reactions. Each vitamin which has particular relevance to the development of pre-menstrual symptoms is described in more detail below.

Vitamin A. This comes in two types: retinol (animal-derived), and beta-carotene (vegetable-derived). Deficiency of vitamin A is very rare indeed, and usually only occurs with a grossly inadequate diet or with severe impairment of digestive function. A lack of vitamin A usually results in an impairment of vision at night, or when in the dark. If deficiencies continue, there are further eye, as well as skin changes.

Recently, a number of studies have demonstrated that either poor intakes of vitamin A, or low blood levels, especially of beta-carotene, are associated with a future increased risk of certain types of cancer, including lung cancer. High intakes of fruit and vegetables rich in vitamin A may thus prove to have a cancer-protective effect.

Vitamin B complex. This is a group of several vitamins with certain things in common. They are all water-soluble, their metabolisms are often inter-related, and they are frequently found together in the same types of foods. Factors that lead to deficiency often, but not always, produce a deficiency of several of the vitamins in this group. Deficiency very often produces mental changes which have many similarities with those of Pre-Menstrual Syndrome.

Vitamin B1, Thiamin, is essential for the normal metabolism of sugar. Requirements for this vitamin increase if the diet is high in sugar, refined carbohydrates and alcohol. Some subtstances which destroy thiamin are found in tea, coffee and raw fish. Good sources of this vitamin are whole-grains, most meats (preferably additive-free or organic) and beans. Any food that is refined is usually quite substantially depleted in thiamin. A lack of thiamin results in anxiety, depression, irritability, changes in behaviour, aggressiveness and loss of memory.

Vitamin B2, Riboflavin, is required for the metabolism of proteins, fats and carbohydrates, particularly in the liver. Deficiency rarely occurs as this vitamin is present in such a wide range of foods, including milk, cheese, meat, fish and some vegetables. Deficiency does not usually produce any mental symptoms. However, vitamin B2 is necessary for the metabolism of vitamin B6 (pyridoxine).

Vitamin B3, Nicotinic Acid or Nicotinamide, is essential for the metabolism of carbohydrates and the release of energy from them. It is found in brown rice, wheatgerm, peanuts and liver. Deficiency rarely occurs unless there is a very poor diet or a high intake of alcohol. In deficiency states, dry scaling and redness appear in light exposed areas, particularly the backs of hands, face, neck and top of the chest. Mental deterioration and diarrhoea are also features, but severe deficiency is very rare. Requirements are between 12 and 15 mg a day. B3 is present in yeast, liver, meat, poultry, legumes, wheat flour and corn. Eggs and milk contain a niacin equivalent called tryptophan.

Vitamin B6 comes in three different varieties: pyridoxine, pyridoxal and pyridoxamine. Pyridoxine is the sort normally used in vitamin supplements, and is also generally used in the treatment of Pre-Menstrual Syndrome. Vitamin B6 requires a supply of vitamin B2 – riboflavin – and magnesium before it is chemically active. Vitamin B6 plays a crucial role in the metabolism of proteins and in the normal metabolism of certain chemicals involved in the brain that control mood and behaviour. Good sources of vitamin B6 include most animal and vegetable proteins, especially fish, egg yolk, wholegrain cereals, nuts and seeds. Bananas, avocados, meat and some green leafy vegetables are also high in this nutrient. A McDonald's Big Mac hamburger contains only 0.02 mg of pyridoxine, which is only 1–2 per cent of that required per day. In fact, it does not contain enough vitamin B6 for the metabolism of the protein contained in the hamburger! Thus a diet containing a significant quantity of such depleted foods, will undoubtedly lead to vitamin B6 deficiency. Other factors which seem to affect it adversely include alcohol and smoking. Deficiency of vitamin B6 produces anxiety, depression, loss of sense of responsibility and insomnia.

Some 15 per cent of women of child-bearing age in the UK have been found to have laboratory evidence of mild vitamin B6 deficiency.

Vitamin B12 and Folic acid. These two types of vitamin B are very important, particularly for the formation of blood and the functioning of nerves. Deficiencies tend to be rare. Vitamin B12 is found almost exclusively in animal produce, especially meat. Long-term vegetarians can be at risk of deficiency unless they take supplements.

Lack of Folic acid can occur from a poor diet, especially if you do not consume plenty of green, leafy vegetables. The name Folic acid comes from foliage, a major source of this important nutrient.

Increased requirements of vitamin B12 and Folic acid occur during pregnancy. Supplements of Folic acid are often given during pregnancy and vitamin B12 should be given to pregnant and breast-feeding mothers if they have been long-term strict vegetarians.

Vitamin C. Almost everyone knows that vitamin C deficiency causes scurvy, and we all think of scurvy as a disease of sailors in the past, and perhaps the extreme deprivation of Victorian times. Indeed, vitamin C deficiency is quite rare but still does occur in some elderly folk. However, in modern times, some people are at risk of having a lower level of vitamin C than is desirable for health. Smoking, in particular, reduces vitamin C levels substantially. The recommended daily intake in this country is only some 40 mg per day, about the amount in an orange.

The increased intake of vitamin C may improve certain aspects of metabolism. In particular, the absorption of iron is helped by the presence of vitamin C in the food. Vitamin C is also necessary for the normal production of sex hormones and the breakdown of excess cholesterol in the body.

Deficiency of vitamin C produces depression, low energy and hypochondria, a condition in which the victim imagines he or she has a variety of different illnesses and complaints. Sometimes, an early sign of vitamin C deficiency is the presence of small pinpoint bruises under the tongue. This seems to be particularly common in smokers.

Vitamin E. Vitamin E is also known as tocopherol, from the Greek words meaning 'child-bearing'. The name is given because rats deprived of vitamin E are unable to bear healthy offspring. Like vitamin C deficiency, vitamin E deficiency is also rare. There are no obvious symptoms or signs of its deficiency, but lack of it is likely to be caused by long-standing digestive problems. Supplements of vitamin E have also been used to treat Pre-Menstrual Syndrome and breast tenderness with some success. It is probable that extra vitamin E is not correcting a deficiency, but improving some aspect of metabolism. The normal daily requirements are in the region of 8–10 mg, which can usually be obtained from dietary sources such as vegetable oils, nuts, green vegetables, eggs and dairy produce.

Like vitamin A, recent evidence has appeared to suggest that low levels of vitamin E in women may be associated with an increased risk of breast cancer in later years. Again, ensuring a good intake of foods rich in such a vitamin may help you achieve good health, not only today, but also for your future tomorrows.

Vitamin D. Vitamin D is necessary for normal healthy bones and teeth. Most of us make adequate vitamin D if our skin is exposed to sunlight. Some can also be provided by the diet as in cod liver oil and dairy produce. Margarine in this country has vitamin D as well as vitamin A added to it. Vitamin D helps the body's absorption of calcium from the diet. In particular, it assists in the normal uptake of calcium into the bones and teeth to make them strong. Too much vitamin D can be toxic, more than 400 international units per day should not be consumed without medical advice.

MINERALS

Minerals are essential components, and may be divided into two types. First there are those minerals which are required in substantial bulk quantities. These include calcium, phosphorus, magnesium, sodium and potassium. They play a large part in the formation of bones and cells. Some other minerals are required in only small amounts and are called trace elements. These include iron, zinc, copper, chromium, selenium and a variety of others. Their main function, like many vitamins, is to help stimulate the complex chemical reactions that take place in the body. A lack of these trace elements, rather like a lack of vitamins, can have a very wide-ranging dire effect upon the body's metabolism. Often the chemical reactions that control energy level and mood, as well as hormone function, can be adversely influenced.

Calcium and Phosphorus. These two minerals often go together, particularly in bones and teeth. It is important to have a good balance of calcium and phosphorus in the diet and the ratio of 2:1 is often recommended. Too much phosphorus will block the absorption of calcium and too much calcium will block the absorption of phosphorus. It is very rare that our diets lack phosphorus, but a lack of calcium is not so uncommon. Good sources of calcium include all dairy products, many nuts, especially Brazils and almonds, bony fish such as sardines, sprats and whitebait, beans, peas, lentils, wholegrains and some green vegetables, especially watercress. In fact, you do not have to eat dairy produce to get an adequate source of calcium but the rest of your diet must be very well balanced indeed. Recommended intakes vary between 700 mg and 1300 mg per day. The absorption of calcium is blocked by bran. Bran contains phytic acid, a substance that combines with calcium, preventing its absorption. (Indian chapattis may also have a similar effect.)

Many convenience foods contain phosphates in the form of food additives: soft drinks, including the low-calorie variety, are notoriously high in phosphate. As a high level interferes with calcium or magnesium balance, these products should be avoided as much as possible.

Magnesium. Magnesium seems to be a particularly important mineral as far as PMS is concerned. Firstly, magnesium, like calcium, is essential for healthy bones as well as nerves and muscles. Lack of magnesium produces poor appetite, nausea, apathy, weakness, tiredness, mood changes and muscle cramps. Good sources of magnesium include most wholefoods, e.g. wholegrains, beans, peas, lentils, nuts, seeds and green vegetables. Water, particularly some bottled waters and tap water from a hard water area, can contain substantial quantities of this mineral, too.

In 1981 Dr Guy Abraham showed that a low level of magnesium was commonly found in women with PMS. Most of the magnesium is inside cells where it is busily involved in chemical reactions. Hence it is the level of magnesium inside the cells – red blood cell magnesium – and not the magnesium in the water compartment of blood that is often low. We repeated his work on magnesium deficiency in 105 women with PMS and showed that some 45 per cent of women had evidence of magnesium deficiency. We don't know precisely how important this deficiency is, but it seems likely that it has an effect on our mental function, the control of the levels of blood sugar and energy, and also the metabolism of some hormones. Unfortunately, there may be no obvious physical signs of magnesium deficiency and so it is easily missed.

Like calcium, requirements increase substantially during pregnancy and while breast-feeding, and it is often after a pregnancy and breast-feeding that the worst cases of magnesium deficiency are seen. This may well explain why some women's pre-menstrual problems begin shortly after childbirth. Indeed, magnesium deficiency is also associated with some other problems such as poor contractions of the womb during labour, elevated blood pressure during pregnancy and pre-eclamptic toxaemia. These conditions can be treated by injections of magnesium, an approach often used in the US, but not so much in the UK.

It is important that women with PMS consume a diet rich in magnesium. Sometimes your doctor can arrange for a simple red cell magnesium test to be performed at the local hospital and this may serve as a guide to the use of magnesium supplements.

Sodium and Potassium. These two minerals form an interesting pair. Both sodium and potassium are essential for the normal functioning of almost all cells in the body, particularly nerves and muscles. Since the use of more convenience foods, our diets have had markedly increased levels of sodium. Although table salt and sea salt (both are sodium chloride) represent a substantial source of sodium in our diets, most of the sodium we consume is found in convenience and other tinned, frozen or prepared foods.

Potassium is found mainly in fruit and vegetables, particularly tomatoes, bananas, figs, citrus fruits and almost all green leafy vegetables. Most of the potassium is found inside the cells rather like magnesium, and most of the sodium is found outside the cells. It is the balance of sodium and potassium that is important. This balance has to be maintained: if it is not, then the body may retain water. Too much sodium in the diet is indeed the commonest cause of fluid retention in many women, particularly in the week or so before the start of a period.

Water tablets, known as diuretics, will get rid of this excess fluid retention, but after a while the system gets used to them and the fluid retention returns, sometimes even worse than before. As well as getting rid of the excess water in the body, diuretics have the effect of ridding the body of useful potassium and magnesium, which makes the situation worse.

The answer: reduce sodium intake in the diet by not having salt at the table, not using it in the cooking, and avoiding any salty foods. It is difficult, on the contrary, to consume too much potassium, and problems only arise in patients with kidney disease.

Iron. Iron is one of the most important trace minerals. We all know that iron is necessary for healthy blood and a lack of it results in anaemia. Iron is necessary for the formation of the blood pigment haemoglobin. What is not widely appreciated is that iron is also found in high concentrations in muscles and in the brain. It is necessary for the uptake of energy by muscles as well as for certain aspects of mental function in the normal brain. Iron deficiency is probably the most common deficiency in the world. Women, of course, have increased needs for iron because of their monthly blood-loss due to menstruation. Women who have heavy periods, such as those using the coil, often have increased requirements.

Good sources of iron include wholefoods such as peas, beans, lentils, nuts, seeds and wholegrains, eggs, meat and to a lesser extent fish. The iron from animal sources is easily absorbed, whereas iron from vegetarian sources may not be so well absorbed, particularly if tea and coffee are consumed at the same meal. Vitamin C in the diet may greatly assist the absorption of iron from vegetarian foods.

The features of iron deficiency include fatigue, tiredness, digestive problems, poor quality nails, and recurrent infections, especially thrush. Although 15 per cent of women of child-bearing age are at risk of developing these problems due to iron deficiency, only one-quarter of these women will actually be anaemic. This means that to detect iron deficiency the doctor must not just measure the haemoglobin level but actually measure the level of iron in the blood for a protein associated with iron called ferritin. If you think you are iron deficient *don't* rely upon your own doctor just doing a test to see if you are anaemic. The iron level or ferritin level must be measured and any deficiency treated. Of course, the most sensible thing to do is to eat a well-balanced diet and avoid the factors that can lead to iron-deficiency. It is a good idea not to drink tea or coffee immediately after meals, but only drink it two hours before or after eating.

Any women with continually heavy periods should have this problem looked into. In fact iron deficiency can even be a cause of heavy periods. Now you can see how important a trace mineral can be!

Zinc. Zinc, like iron, affects many different aspects of metabolism, particularly those involved in growth, and resistance to infection. It is necessary for healthy skin, normal hormone production and normal mental function. Adequate quantities can be obtained from wholegrains, nuts, peas, beans, lentils and meat. Like iron, zinc absorption may be blocked by tea and coffee as the tannin from the drink binds with it, preventing its absorption. You know what strong tea can do to the inside of a white teacup – imagine what it does to the inside of your intestines!

Anyone regularly consuming substantial quantities of alcohol, i.e. more than two glasses of wine or a pint of beer per day, is at risk of developing zinc as well as vitamin B deficiencies. Women on the Pill can have lower levels of zinc, as can those who make long-term use of diuretics – water pills. Often a useful clue to a lack of zinc is poor quality skin such as excessively dry or greasy facial skin, particularly at the sides of the nose. Eczema, acne and psoriasis may also suggest a deficiency of this important mineral. Interestingly, the metabolism of zinc and vitamin B6 are closely related, which explains why the skin changes produced by these two deficiencies can have a similar appearance.

Chromium. Chromium is a fascinating trace mineral. Only minute quantities are required: a lifetime's supply of chromium only weighs one-sixth of an ounce (5 g), and the body will only use 1 per cent of that. Yet even this tiny amount of chromium plays a crucial part in the control of blood sugar metabolism. A lack of chromium can lead to poor blood-sugar control, which in turn can lead to fluctuating energy levels and the dreaded sugar cravings. They are a classic feature of some women's pre-menstrual symptoms, as we have seen.

In severe cases of chromium deficiency a diabetes-like state can occur, particularly in older people. Chromium supplements can have a marked effect in this situation, and can also help improve poor blood-sugar control in people who are not diabetics. Eating large quantities of carbohydrates such as table sugar increases the loss of chromium in the urine. There are no outward signs of chromium deficiency, unless you count the presence of old sweet wrappers in the bottom of your handbag! We have seen no end of 'little miracles' as a result of increasing chromium intake: it really is very useful in helping to control the sugar cravings. Eating a sensible diet is the best way to prevent chromium deficiency. Foods which contain a good quantity of chromium are green vegetables, root vegetables, eggs, scallops, shrimps, rye and some fruit.

That ends all you really need to know about vitamins and minerals. It may be useful to summarize this vital information and indicate how you can recognize any deficiencies.

As a general rule vitamin and mineral deficiencies are caused by a poor diet or the presence in the diet of agents such as alcohol, tea, coffee, cigarettes, poor-quality food, or an excessive consumption of refined carbohydrates. These increase the need for nutrients from the remaining healthy foods that are consumed. If you have any symptoms or signs of deficiencies which persist despite a healthy diet, or despite taking nutritional supplements for a period of three months, then it is important to consult your medical practitioner. In the Self-Help section on diet, beginning on page 147, more attention will be given to the foods which are high in essential vitamins and minerals and how to have a diet with sufficient quantities of each.

VITAMINS AND MINERALS –
DO YOU LACK THEM?

	Food Sources	What They Do
Vitamin B6	Meat, fish, nuts, bananas, avocados, wholegrains	Essential in the metabolism of protein and the amino acids that control mood and behaviour. Affects hormone metabolism
Vitamin B1 Thiamin	Meat, fish, nuts, wholegrains and fortified breakfast cereals	Essential in the metabolism of sugar, especially in nerves and muscles
Vitamin C Ascorbic acid	Any fresh fruits and vegetables	Involved in healing, repair of tissues and production of some hormones
Iron	Meat, wholegrains, nuts, eggs and fortified breakfast cereals	Essential to make blood haemoglobin. Many other tissues need iron for energy reactions
Zinc	Meat, wholegrains, nuts, peas, beans, lentils	Essential for normal growth, mental function, hormone production and resistance to infection
Magnesium	Green vegetables, wholegrains, Brazil and almond nuts, many other non-junk foods	Essential for sugar and energy metabolism, needed for healthy nerves and muscles
Calcium	Milk, cheese, bread, especially white, sardines, other fish with bones, green vegetables and beans	Needed for strong teeth and bones, also for normal nerve and muscle function. Lack leads to osteoporosis – bone thinning
Essential fatty acids – Omega 3	Cod liver oil, mackerel, herring	Help control inflammation
Fish and related oils	Salmon, rape seed and soy bean oil	Reduce calcium losses in urine
Essential fatty acids – Omega 6 evening primrose and related oil	Sunflower, safflower and corn oils, many nuts (not peanuts) and seeds, green vegetables	Control inflammation, needed for health of nervous system, skin and blood vessels

Deficiencies

Who is at Risk	Symptoms	Visible Signs
Women, especially smokers, 'junk-eaters'	Depression, anxiety, insomnia, loss of responsibility	Dry/greasy facial skin, cracking at corners of the mouth
Alcohol consumers, women on the Pill, breast-feeding mothers, high consumers of sugar	Depression, anxiety, poor appetite, nausea, personality change	None usually! Heart, nerve and muscle problems if severe
Smokers particularly	Lethargy, depression hypochondriasis (imagined illnesses)	Easy bruising, look for small pinpoint bruises under the tongue
Women who have heavy periods (e.g. coil users), vegetarians, especially if tea or coffee drinkers, women with recurrent thrush	Fatigue, poor energy, depression, poor digestion, sore tongue, cracking at corners of mouth	Pale complexion, brittle nails, cracking at corners of mouth
Vegetarians, especially tea and coffee drinkers, alcohol consumers, long-term users of diuretics (water pills)	Poor mental function, skin problems in general, repeated infections	Eczema, acne, greasy or dry facial skin
Women with PMS! (some 50 per cent may be lacking), long-term diuretic users, alcohol consumers	Nausea, apathy, loss of appetite, depression, mood changes, muscle cramps	Usually NONE! so easily missed; muscle spasms sometimes
Low dairy consumers, heavy drinkers, smokers, women with early menopause, lack of exercise increases the rate of bone loss-calcium in later years	Usually none until osteoporotic fracture of hip or spine. Back pain	Loss of height
Those on a poor diet	None	None
Older people, diabetics, drinkers	None	None
Those on a poor diet, diabetics and drinkers. Also those with severe eczema and premenstrual breast tenderness	None	Possibly dry skin

TRIED AND TESTED

The value of the nutritional approach to PMS can be measured in a laboratory. Here are three examples of patients who had 'before' and 'after' laboratory tests. These tests allow us to measure vitamin and mineral levels to verify precise deficiencies which can then be treated.

GERALDINE ELLIS

Geraldine had mainly been troubled by PMS D, and episodes of recurrent thrush. In the past, taking the oral contraceptive pill had aggravated her thrush and worsened her feelings of depression, but stopping the Pill had not stopped the thrush. Similarly, nutritional deficiencies can pre-dispose to thrush, especially a deficiency of iron, and Geraldine was quite severely iron-deficient. The level of iron in her blood was 2 micromols per litre, normal range being 11–29. She was iron-deficient even though she was not anaemic. Iron is necessary, not just for making the blood pigment haemoglobin, but also because it helps to strengthen muscles and improves the digestive system and the ability of cells to fight infection.

Treatment with supplements of iron, multi-vitamins and a further course of anti-fungal treatment to control her thrush resulted in a substantial improvement in Geraldine's pre-menstrual symptoms, clearance of her thrush and correction of the iron deficiency itself. She also had a low level of magnesium in the red cells so required an additional magnesium supplement.

SANDRA PATTERSON

Sandra was a 29-year-old, single girl for whom Pre-Menstrual Syndrome carried a very special significance: on two occasions pre-menstrually she had inadvertently shoplifted. In her pre-menstrual confusion she had forgotten to pay for goods as she left the shop. The mistake was picked up by the store detective before she herself had time to return to the shop and pay for them. The courts put her on probation the first time and Sandra decided she must do something about the Pre-Menstrual Syndrome. She started taking Efamol evening primrose oil, 500 mg capsules, four per day. This controlled her pre-menstrual symptoms extremely well, so well in fact that after a few months she stopped them altogether. Unfortunately, the next month her PMS returned and with it her second shoplifting episode. The court was now beginning to find her story hard to believe.

In fact, the laboratory investigations showed that Sandra had some marked nutritional deficiencies of zinc and vitamin B6. The activity of vitamin B6 in her blood was 46 per cent below an optimum level, the normal range being up to 15 per cent below – this indicated a severe deficiency. Similarly, the level of zinc was also depressed by some 25 per cent. Both zinc and vitamin B6 deficiencies may have influenced mental function and mood. Both play a crucial part in the metabolism of essential fatty acids, a specialized form of which is found in evening primrose oil. Thus it was that evening primrose oil was controlling Sandra's symptoms, without correcting all the underlying nutritional deficiencies. When an appropriate supplement of zinc and vitamin B6 was combined with her evening primrose oil, her pre-menstrual symptoms once again disappeared completely. With a better diet she was able to reduce her need for nutritional supplements. Fortunately the court took a lenient attitude on the second occasion, and she is now well aware of the responsibility she has to look after herself.

REBECCA HARLEY

Rebecca had a long history of Pre-Menstrual Syndrome and low energy levels which showed a significant improvement when her nutritional problems were treated. Investigations showed her to have a very low level of magnesium. The red cell value was 1.5 millimols per litre, normal range being 2–3. Treatment with magnesium supplements, multi-vitamins (especially vitamin B6) and avoiding salt and wheat, made a substantial reduction in her symptoms of PMS H, fluid retention, abdominal bloating, as well as her other symptoms of anxiety, depression and fatigue. However, the fatigue was persistent and she had a rather puffy facial appearance. This suggested that the thyroid gland might be underactive. First tests were normal, but repeat tests a few months later showed that the thyroid was indeed beginning to fail. The pituitary gland, at the base of the brain, normally produces a thyroid stimulation hormone known as TSH. The TSH level had increased to 5.2 micro units per litre, when the normal value should be less than 5. Thus the pituitary gland was producing slightly increased amounts of hormone to try to stimulate the failing thyroid. Treatment with small quantities of thyroid hormone made a dramatic difference to Rebecca's symptoms. Initially, her magnesium level rose to 2.55 millimols per litre, thus showing full correction of the deficiency. An underactive thyroid should always be considered in women with Pre-Menstrual Syndrome, especially PMS H symptoms which do not respond to other treatment. An underactive thyroid may be the underlying cause not only of PMS, but also of heavy periods, a lack of periods, weight gain, decreased energy level, depression, mental sluggishness and dry skin.

RESULTS OF THE WOMEN'S NUTRITIONAL ADVISORY SERVICE PROGRAMME FOR PMS

Over the years the WNAS has conducted a number of studies to assess the value of the WNAS programme. The two most important questions that we have tried to answer are: *How easy or difficult is the programme to follow,* and *How successful is it?*

The first study we conducted was in 1985. Looking at 382 women who were sent a postal programme, we found that at least 245 of them followed the programme either completely or to a reasonable degree. Thus we knew that at least two-thirds of women found the programme acceptable. Further analysis showed that the more closely the programme was followed the more successful the outcome. In those who followed it completely (150 women) 91 per cent of the symptoms marked as severe in the pre-menstrual week reduced to either none, mild or moderate. Overall, 87 per cent of these women felt that they had benefited considerably by three months.

Of the 150 women, 93 were already taking other treatment for their PMS, usually vitamin B6 alone, hormonal treatments, diuretics or anti-depressants. Seventy-five per cent of these 93 women were able to stop all their previous treatment, 16 per cent reduced the dosage and 9 per cent continued unchanged.

In 1988 we looked at a further group of 200 women who had completed all their questionnaires on the postal programme. Again, the degree of improvement depended very much on how closely the programme was followed, particularly for the dietary side of their treatment. Ninety-six per cent of those who had followed the programme reported that they were significantly better within the first three months. We also found that women who were overweight lost between eight and 13 pounds, depending on how large they were to start with, without trying! It is now known that even modest weight loss in those who are overweight and have period problems can have a powerful corrective effect on hormonal abnor-malities.

In 1990 we conducted a survey of 100 women who began the postal pro-gramme and we tried to contact them all so that we had as true a result as possible about the results of the programme. We were able to contact 88 of the 100 women. Sixty-nine of them had followed the programme. The reasons why the others had not were: pregnancy, other illnesses such as appendicitis, family stress including divorce and a death in the family, or because the programme was considered too difficult. This last was the case for 10 women. So we knew from this that the programme could be followed by some 70 per cent of women and that the success rate in them was also about 70 per cent. This compared very favourably with the outcome of most drug and hormone trials on PMS.

We tried to learn some lessons from these studies. Firstly, we realized that we had to be as scientific as possible about the supplements, and for many years we have limited our use to those preparations that are scientifically proven to be of value in PMS. Secondly, the diet has to be as easy as possible whilst still being thorough, and this means giving a good number of alternatives. This has become much easier over the years as caffeine-free, salt-free, low-fat foods have appeared on the supermarket shelves. Finally, the better the support from the WNAS the better the degree of improvement.

It was also obvious to us that there will always be some women whom we will be unable to help. As I have said elsewhere, certain medical and gynaecological problems can cause PMS, which will not fully improve until the problems themselves are corrected. We now include a number of questions on our questionnaire to try and identify those who would be well advised to have a gynaecological check.

We did a further analysis of those women who attended our clinics in London and Sussex during 1992. These women received detailed, tailor-made advice about their diets with many diet sheets and sample menus, advice about nutritional supplements, some of which were prescribable by their GPs, and advice to exercise. Every effort was made to help women make the necessary changes to their diets. Each woman who attended one of the clinics was either seen again or reported on their progress by telephone. The minimum duration for assessment was two months and most were assessed at three or four months.

Out of a total of 75 women, two women who attended did not actually have PMS but had depression that lasted throughout the month, and they were referred back to their family doctor. The remaining 73 were considered to have moderate to severe PMS and they were all given appropriate advice. Within the first week, two of the women considered that the diet was too difficult for them to follow because of their lifestyles. They both travelled extensively and ate almost all their meals away from home. A further two women could not be contacted because they had moved or were travelling abroad.

This left 69 women, two of whom became pregnant within the first month and were thus excluded from the analysis. (Pregnancy is not a side-effect of the programme!) All of them were asked to complete detailed questionnaires detailing the severity of their symptoms and the degree to which they followed the programme. We found that 97 per cent of the women had complied with the recommendations made, and 76 per cent were significantly better after an average of three to four months. We found that their home life had improved by 72 per cent, work efficiency by 62 per cent, sexual relationship by 50 per cent (enjoyment of sex by 36 per cent and frequency by 32 per cent). Improvements in violent behaviour amounted to 60 per cent, aches and pains by 43 per cent, driving ability by 47 per cent, concentration by 54 per cent and confusion by 59 per cent. These improved compliance figures almost certainly reflect the greater degree of co-operation that can be achieved in a clinic setting than with a postal programme, and also refinements made to the programme over the years. When we looked further at the relationship between the degree of success and the degree of adherence to the different parts of the programme, again we found that the best improvement was obtained in those who followed the programme most carefully, especially the dietary side.

Only one of the women needed to take a drug, an anti-depressant, because of severe depression in addition to her PMS. Four of the 69 women were also found to have other health problems that had not been previously investigated, and these were: repeated miscarriages, deafness due to a hormone sensitivity, a hormone abnormality related to ovarian cysts, and some unusual food intolerances. All such women needed to be referred to their GP and on to a specialist for further assessment and treatment. Sometimes, therefore, PMS may mask other conditions that require treatment in their own right.

The overall message, I am delighted to say, is that it is a very effective programmme, and that not only does it help to overcome the majority of PMS symptoms, it also provides an education about diet, and a getting-to-know-what-your-body-likes-and-dislikes process, which most of us have missed out on in the past. Energy levels improve, women experience a great sense of well-being, and it has a wonderful knock-on effect for the husbands and children, both in dietary and social terms.

PART THREE

THE NUTRITIONAL
APPROACH – A SELF-
HELP MANUAL

15

CHOOSING A NUTRITIONAL PLAN

The Nutritional Approach to PMS is one which involves making dietary and lifestyle changes. It may span a very broad spectrum, in that mild sufferers only need to make a few dietary changes, whilst the moderate and severe sufferers need to follow a more specialized diet and perhaps even change their lifestyle to some degree.

In order to accommodate all PMS sufferers, I have prepared three options for you to choose from:

Option 1 Basic dietary and health recommendations – for mild sufferers.

Option 2 A specialized dietary plan – for moderate sufferers.

Option 3 A tailor-made nutritional programme – for moderate and severe sufferers.

Be guided by the severity of symptoms when making your choice of option, and not the convenience of one regime as opposed to another!

The closer you stick to the recommendations, the better your chances of rapid improvement. It's worth bearing this in mind as you go along, especially if you find it hard going making some of the changes.

OPTION 1 – BASIC DIETARY AND HEALTH RECOMMENDATIONS

1. **Reduce intake of sugar and 'junk' foods.** This includes sugar added to tea and coffee, sweets, cakes, chocolates, biscuits, puddings, jams, marmalade, soft drinks, ice cream and honey. Consumption of these

foods may cause water retention and block the uptake of essential minerals.

2. **Reduce intake of salt, both added during the cooking and at the table.** Also reduce the intake of salty foods, e.g. salted nuts, kippers, bacon, etc. This causes fluid retention and may contribute to other PMS symptoms.

3. **Reduce intake of tea and coffee.** Consume no more than one or two cups of tea and coffee per day. There are many pleasant herbal teas and substitutes for coffee from healthfood shops.

4. **Eat green vegetables or salad daily.** A good helping of either of these should be obtained and eaten every day. Both of these contain important vitamins and minerals useful in the treatment of PMS symptoms.

5. **Limit your intake of dairy products.** Have at least two good servings of dairy products per day, apart from milk used in drinks. Have milk and/or yoghurt with your cereal and another serving of yoghurt or cheese each day, unless you have a sensitivity to dairy products.

6. **Reduce intake of tobacco and alcohol.** These aggravate some PMS symptoms.

7. **Use good vegetable oils.** A good-quality vegetable oil, such as sunflower or safflower seed oil, should be used for any cooking, or for making salad dressings. Similarly, a sunflower seed margarine should be used rather than butter or other margarine.

8. **Eat plenty of wholefoods.** By 'wholefoods' we mean foods, usually of vegetable origin, which have not been processed or refined, e.g. wholemeal bread and cereals, such as rye, oats, barley and millet. Food such as nuts and seeds are high in vitamins and minerals as too are the important vegetable oils. If eating meat, make sure that it is lean, and eat fish and poultry too. Certain fish, e.g. herring and salmon, contain some essential oils which are helpful in maintaining skin quality and may be of some value in preventing pre-menstrual breast tenderness.

9. **Have regular exercise.** Physical exercise is of proven value in the treatment of pre-menstrual symptoms. Certainly those with a sedentary

job, particularly those who do not get into the fresh air, should take regular physical exercise. Exercise, fresh air and exposure to sunlight are important factors in maintaining health, just as important as ensuring a healthy diet and taking vitamin and mineral supplements.

10. **Take a walk.** In moments of pure desperation or impending aggression, please do immediately take a walk. Get out of the house and change your environment. Walk quietly, taking notice of the things around you. Do this until you feel a bit better.

OPTION 2 – A SPECIALIZED DIETARY PLAN

As well as following the broad dietary recommendations outlined in Option 1 you will need to select a diet that will help your particular symptoms. Once you have worked out which vitamins and minerals you need to concentrate on from the chart below, you can then go on to refer to the food lists and menus that apply to you.

BROAD DIETARY REQUIREMENTS FOR PMS AND OTHER RELATED SYMPTOMS

PMS A – nervous tension, mood swings, irritability and anxiety. Sufferers need high vitamin B6 and magnesium diets.

PMS H – weight gain, swelling of extremities, breast tenderness and abdominal bloating. Sufferers need high vitamin E, vitamin B6 and magnesium diets.

PMS C – headache, craving for sweets, increased appetite, heart pounding, fatigue and dizziness or fainting. Sufferers need high vitamin B6, magnesium and chromium diets.

PMS D – depression, forgetfulness, crying, confusion and insomnia. Sufferers need high vitamin B6, magnesium and vitamin C diets.

Acne/skin problems. A diet high in zinc is needed.

Smokers. Need high vitamin C diets.

Anaemic/heavy periods. Need high iron diets.

If, for example, you decide you are suffering with PMS A (Anxiety) and PMS C (Sugar Cravings) you will need to concentrate on a diet high in vitamin B6, magnesium and chromium. You simply refer to the relevant food lists on pages 155–163 when selecting the foods to include in your daily diet. I have also prepared a sample daily menu (see below) plus a sample menu plan for one week. These are designed to give you a guide to balanced menu planning. They are not something you have to follow, but you might like to use them as a starting point.

WHERE TO SHOP

I will be suggesting that you eat plenty of salads, vegetables and fruit. You will have realized from Chapter 11 in Part Two that many of these foods are contaminated with chemicals. While many of the large supermarkets now stock organic produce it is usually only a limited range. Although a little more expensive, if you can possibly manage to buy it, you'll be better off. That is, unless you have a local organic farm or grow your own organic produce, which makes even more sense.

Whilst there are many vegetarian suggestions and recipes included, I have catered for meat- and fish-eaters as well. Again, because of the chemicals and drugs in meat, I would suggest you try to find a butcher who will buy additive-free meat for you from an organic farm.

Changing over to a full range of organic produce is going to take some time. Currently the demands by retailers for organic produce cannot be met. As more and more farmers switch, there will hopefully be plenty to go round.

SAMPLE DAILY MENU

Breakfast

Muesli *or* an oat crunchy cereal with a piece of chopped fruit (e.g. a banana, some grapes, berries, etc.)
with milk or yoghurt

Followed by:
One or two slices of wholemeal toast *or* rye crispbread
with low sugar jam or marmalade

Alternatively:
2 scrambled eggs or omelette with grilled tomatoes and mushrooms
or boiled or poached eggs
Wholemeal toast or rye crispbread and low sugar spreads

Mid-morning snack

See **Snack list** below.

Lunch

Cold meat *or* fresh or tinned fish with salad platter or sandwiches
or
Pasta and vegetables
or
Jacket potato with a nutritious filling – for example:
  Tuna and sweetcorn with a little sour cream and black pepper
  Prawns
  Baked beans
  Curried chicken
or
Home-made soup and salad and wholemeal bread or rye crispbread

Tea-time snack

See **Snack list** below.

Dinner

Poultry/fish/meat or vegetarian protein served with three portions of
vegetables.
Fresh fruit or a fresh fruit salad
or
choose an appropriate sweet from the dessert section or from the *Beat PMS
Cookbook*

Snack list

Rye crispbread and fruit spreads or peanut butter
Jordan's 'Fruesli' bar or oat crunchy bars
Scones and low sugar jam
Pasta or bean salad

Corn chips or papadoms made from dhal flour
Raw vegetables and dips like hummus, taramasalata or guacamole
Fresh fruit, nuts *or* seeds
Yoghurt and fruit

Beverages

Coffee substitutes. Barley Cup, Caro, Bambu, dandelion coffee, chicory, or up to two cups of decaffeinated coffee per day.

Herbal teas. Rooibosch Eleven O'clock tea (with milk). This herbal tea 'look alike', available from healthfood shops, contains a mild, natural muscle relaxant and may help alleviate tension and ease period pains. It is favoured by many of our patients and is definitely worth a try. Other suggestions are bramble, raspberry and ginseng, mixed berry, lemon verbena, fennel and wild strawberry. These days most healthfood shops sell single sachets so that you can 'buy and try' without being saddled with a whole box of tea bags that you absolutely detest.

Cold drinks. Bottled water with or without fruit juice, mineral water, Appletise, Aqua Libra, or Irish Spring or Amé.

OPTION 2 – FAST OPTION LUNCHES

Have a salad with:
  Cheese omelette
  Jacket potato with tuna, sweetcorn, margarine, cheese or beans
  Sardines on toast
  Nut butter sandwich with fruit salad
  French stick with mackerel and salad
  Scrambled egg
  Beans on toast
  Prepared pasta such as ravioli or tortellini
  Avocado pear
  Chicken, turkey or fish
  Raw vegetable crudité, corn chips and dips such as hummus, taramasalata or guacamole
  Fresh fruit, nuts and yoghurt
  Pitta bread with prawns, chicken or fish
  Danish open sandwich or pumpernickel

OPTION 2 – FAST OPTION DINNERS

Have three portions of vegetables, including a green leafy vegetable with:
Grilled sardines with a jacket potato
Poached salmon
Kangaroo steak and chips
Stir-fry vegetables with nuts, beans, Quorn, prawns or chicken and rice
or noodles
Potato bake
Tofu burgers and salad
Grilled lamb chop
Mackerel coated in rolled oats and grilled with salad
Lasagne
Fish pie
Prawn and egg salad
Wholemeal pancakes with vegetables and cheese sauce
Cauliflower and broccoli cheese with a jacket potato
Mixed bean salad with hummus and pitta bread

A SAMPLE MENU PLAN FOR ONE WEEK

See above for **Beverages**. As your calorie requirements increase by up to
500 calories per day in the pre-menstrual week, make sure you have a mid-
morning and mid-afternoon snack each day of that week in order to keep
your blood sugar levels constant. (See **Snack list** on page 151.)

B = Breakfast   L = Lunch   D = Dinner   S = Sweet
Recipes in Chapter 17, page 208.

DAY 1
B   Orange juice
    Muesli (home-made) with
      milk
L   Broccoli soup
    1 slice of wholemeal
      (wholewheat) bread
D   Mackerel with herbs (foil-
      baked)
    Brown rice salad
    Apple and celery salad

S   Baked pears with raisins

DAY 2
B   Fresh grapefruit and orange
      salad with sunflower seeds
    Toast and dried fruit conserve
      or sugar-free jam (jelly)
L   Stuffed peppers (bell peppers)
    Banana
D   Roast chicken
    Cabbage

Turnips
Swede (rutabaga) and carrot
  mix
Sliced fried potatoes
S Slice of date and walnut cake

DAY 3

B Apple juice
Poached egg and toast
L Lentil and vegetable soup
Avocado with crab meat or
  prawns (shrimps)
Green bean salad
Fresh orange
D Lamb paprika
Brown rice
S Stuffed baked apple

DAY 4

B Wholewheat pancakes
  (crêpes)
½ quantity dried fruit conserve
½ grapefruit
L Jacket potatoes with tuna
Bulgar (cracked wheat) and
  nut salad
Orange and cucumber salad
Slice of melon
D Steamed fish with garlic,
  spring (green) onions and
  ginger
Stir-fried vegetables
S Rhubarb fool

DAY 5

B Orange juice
Scrambled eggs and tomatoes
  with toast

L Grilled sardines
1 slice wholemeal
  (wholewheat) bread
Beanshoot salad
Grapes
2 slices of rye crackers
D Nut roast
Brown rice
Waldorf salad
S Fresh fruit salad

DAY 6

B Grapefruit juice
Yoghurt with sliced apple and
  raisins
L Nutty parsnip soup
Cheese omelette
Red cabbage, apple and bean
  salad
Plums
D Liver with orange
Leafy green vegetables
Boiled potatoes
Cauliflower and carrots
S Ginger bananas

DAY 7

B Apple juice
Poached haddock
Tomatoes and mushrooms
L Cauliflower and leeks in
  cheese sauce
Slice of bread
Orange
D Vegetarian goulash
Brown rice
S Fresh fruit salad

NUTRITIONAL CONTENT OF FOOD

Unless stated otherwise, foods listed are raw

VITAMIN A – RETINOL
Micrograms per 100 g (3.5 oz)

Skimmed milk	1
Semi-skimmed milk	21
Grilled herring	49
Whole milk	52
Porridge made with milk	56
Cheddar cheese	325
Margarine	800
Butter	815
Lamb's liver	15,000

VITAMIN B1 – THIAMIN
Milligrams per 100 g (3.5 oz)

Peaches	0.02
Cottage cheese	0.02
Cox's apple	0.03
Full-fat milk	0.04
Skimmed milk	0.04
Semi-skimmed milk	0.04
Cheddar cheese	0.04
Bananas	0.04
White grapes	0.04
French beans	0.04
Low-fat yoghurt	0.05
Cantaloupe melon	0.05
Tomato	0.06
Green peppers, raw	0.07
Boiled egg	0.08
Roast chicken	0.08
Grilled cod	0.08
Haddock, steamed	0.08
Roast turkey	0.09
Mackerel, cooked	0.09
Savoy cabbage, boiled	0.10
Oranges	0.10
Brussels sprouts	0.10
Lentils, boiled	0.11
Potatoes, new, boiled	0.11
Soya beans, boiled	0.12
Red peppers, raw	0.12
Lentils, boiled	0.14
Steamed salmon	0.20
Corn	0.20
White spaghetti, boiled	0.21
Almonds	0.24
White self-raising flour	0.30
Plaice, steamed	0.30
Bacon, cooked	0.35
Walnuts	0.40
Wholemeal flour	0.47
Lamb's kidney	0.49
Brazil nuts	1.00
Cornflakes	1.00
Rice Krispies	1.00
Wheatgerm	2.01

VITAMIN B2 – RIBOFLAVIN
Milligrams per 100 g (3.5 oz)

Cabbage, boiled	0.01
Potatoes, boiled	0.01
Brown rice, boiled	0.02
Pear	0.03
Wholemeal spaghetti, boiled	0.03
White self-raising flour	0.03
Orange	0.04
Spinach, boiled in salted water	0.05
Baked beans	0.06
Banana	0.06
White bread	0.06
Green peppers, raw	0.08
Lentils, boiled	0.08
Hovis	0.09

Food	mg	Food	mg
Soya beans, boiled	0.09	Avocado	1.10
Wholemeal bread	0.09	Green peppers, raw	1.10
Wholemeal flour	0.09	Brown rice	1.30
Peanuts	0.10	Wholemeal spaghetti, boiled	1.30
Baked salmon	0.11	White self-raising flour	1.50
Red peppers, raw	0.15	Grilled cod	1.70
Full-fat milk	0.17	White bread	1.70
Avocado	0.18	Soya flour	2.00
Grilled herring	0.18	Red peppers, raw	2.20
Semi-skimmed milk	0.18	Almonds	3.10
Roast chicken	0.19	Grilled herring	4.00
Roast turkey	0.21	Wholemeal bread	4.10
Cottage cheese	0.26	Hovis	4.20
Soya flour	0.31	Wholemeal flour	5.70
Boiled prawns	0.34	Muesli	6.50
Boiled egg	0.35	Topside of beef, cooked	6.50
Topside of beef, cooked	0.35	Leg of lamb, cooked	6.60
Leg of lamb, cooked	0.38	Baked salmon	7.00
Cheddar cheese	0.40	Roast chicken	8.20
Muesli	0.70	Roast turkey	8.50
Almonds	0.75	Boiled prawns	9.50
Cornflakes	1.50	Peanuts	13.80
Rice Krispies	1.50	Cornflakes	16.00
		Rice Krispies	16.00

VITAMIN B3 – NIACIN
Milligrams per 100 g (3.5 oz)

Food	mg
Boiled egg	0.07
Cheddar cheese	0.07
Full-fat milk	0.08
Skimmed milk	0.09
Semi-skimmed milk	0.09
Cottage cheese	0.13
Cox's apple	0.20
Cabbage, boiled	0.30
Orange	0.40
Baked beans	0.50
Potatoes, boiled	0.50
Soya beans, boiled	0.50
Lentils, boiled	0.60
Banana	0.70
Tomato	1.00

VITAMIN B6 – PYRIDOXINE
Milligrams per 100 g (3.5 oz)

Food	mg
Carrots	0.05
Full-fat milk	0.06
Skimmed milk	0.06
Semi-skimmed milk	0.06
Satsuma	0.07
White bread	0.07
White rice	0.07
Cabbage, boiled	0.08
Cottage cheese	0.08
Cox's apple	0.08
Wholemeal pasta	0.08
Frozen peas	0.09
Spinach, boiled	0.09
Cheddar cheese	0.10

Orange	0.10	Semi-skimmed milk	0.40
Broccoli	0.11	Marmite	0.50
Hovis	0.11	Cottage cheese	0.70
Baked beans	0.12	Choux buns	1.00
Boiled egg	0.12	Eggs, boiled	1.00
Red kidney beans, cooked	0.12	Eggs, poached	1.00
Wholemeal bread	0.12	Halibut, steamed	1.00
Tomatoes	0.14	Lobster, boiled	1.00
Almonds	0.15	Sponge cake	1.00
Cauliflower	0.15	Turkey, white meat	1.00
Brussels sprouts	0.19	Waffles	1.00
Sweetcorn, boiled	0.21	Cheddar cheese	1.20
Leg of lamb, cooked	0.22	Eggs, scrambled	1.20
Grapefruit juice	0.23	Squid	1.30
Roast chicken	0.26	Eggs, fried	1.60
Lentils, boiled	0.28	Shrimps, boiled	1.80
Banana	0.29	Parmesan cheese	1.90
Brazil nuts	0.31	Beef, lean	2.00
Potatoes, boiled	0.32	Cod, baked	2.00
Roast turkey	0.33	Cornflakes	2.00
Grilled herring	0.33	Pork, cooked	2.00
Topside of beef, cooked	0.33	Raw beef mince	2.00
Avocado	0.36	Rice Krispies	2.00
Grilled cod	0.38	Steak, lean, grilled	2.00
Baked salmon	0.57	Edam cheese	2.10
Soya flour	0.57	Eggs, whole, battery	2.40
Hazelnuts	0.59	Milk, dried, whole	2.40
Peanuts	0.59	Milk, dried skimmed	2.60
Walnuts	0.67	Eggs, whole, free-range	2.70
Muesli	1.60	Kambu seaweed	2.80
Cornflakes	1.80	Squid, frozen	2.90
Rice Krispies	1.80	Taramasalata	2.90
Special K	2.20	Duck, cooked	3.00
		Turkey, dark meat	3.00
VITAMIN B12		Grapenuts	5.00
Micrograms per 100 g (3.5 oz)		Tuna in oil	5.00
		Herring, cooked	6.00
		Herring roe, fried	6.00
Tempeh	0.10	Steamed salmon	6.00
Miso	0.20	Bovril	8.30
Quorn	0.30	Mackerel, fried	10.00
Full-fat milk	0.40	Rabbit, stewed	10.00
Skimmed milk	0.40		

Cod's roe, fried	11.00	Cottage cheese	27.00
Pilchards, canned in tomato		Baked salmon	29.00
juice	12.00	Cabbage, boiled	29.00
Oysters, raw	15.00	Onions, boiled	29.00
Nori seaweed	27.50	White bread	29.00
Sardines in oil	28.00	Orange	31.00
Lamb's kidney, fried	79.00	Baked beans	33.00
		Cheddar cheese	33.00

FOLATE/FOLIC ACID
Micrograms per 100 g (3.5 oz)

		Clementines	33.00
		Raspberries	33.00
		Satsuma	33.00
Cox's apple	4.00	Blackberries	34.00
Leg of lamb, cooked	4.00	Rye crispbread	35.00
Full-fat milk	6.00	Potato, baked in skin	36.00
Skimmed milk	6.00	Radish	38.00
Semi-skimmed milk	6.00	Boiled egg	39.00
Porridge with semi-skimmed		Hovis	39.00
milk	7.00	Wholemeal bread	39.00
Turnip, baked	8.00	Red kidney beans, boiled	42.00
Sweet potato, boiled	8.00	Potato, baked	44.00
Cucumber	9.00	Frozen peas	47.00
Grilled herring	10.00	Almonds	48.00
Roast chicken	10.00	Parsnips, boiled	48.00
Avocado	11.00	Cauliflower	51.00
Grilled cod	12.00	Green beans, boiled	57.00
Banana	14.00	Broccoli	64.00
Roast turkey	15.00	Walnuts	66.00
Carrots	17.00	Artichoke	68.00
Sweet potato	17.00	Hazelnuts	72.00
Tomatoes	17.00	Spinach, boiled	90.00
Topside of beef, cooked	17.00	Brussels sprouts	110.00
Swede, boiled	18.00	Peanuts	110.00
Strawberries	20.00	Muesli	140.00
Brazil nuts	21.00	Sweetcorn, boiled	150.00
Red peppers, raw	21.00	Asparagus	155.00
Green peppers, raw	23.00	Chickpeas	180.00
Rye bread	24.00	Lamb's liver, fried	240.00
Dates, fresh	25.00	Cornflakes	250.00
New potatoes, boiled	25.00	Rice Krispies	250.00
Grapefruit	26.00	Calf's liver, fried	320.00
Oatcakes	26.00		

VITAMIN C
Milligrams per 100 g (3.5 oz)

Full-fat milk	1.00
Skimmed milk	1.00
Semi-skimmed milk	1.00
Red kidney beans	1.00
Carrots	2.00
Cucumber	2.00
Muesli with dried fruit	2.00
Apricots, raw	6.00
Avocado	6.00
Pear	6.00
Potato, boiled	6.00
Spinach, boiled	8.00
Cox's apple	9.00
Turnip	10.00
Banana	11.00
Frozen peas	12.00
Lamb's liver, fried	12.00
Pineapple	12.00
Dried skimmed milk	13.00
Gooseberries	14.00
Raw dates	14.00
Melon	17.00
Tomatoes	17.00
Cabbage, boiled	20.00
Cantaloupe melon	26.00
Cauliflower	27.00
Satsuma	27.00
Peach	31.00
Raspberries	32.00
Bran flakes	35.00
Grapefruit	36.00
Mangoes	37.00
Nectarine	37.00
Kumquats	39.00
Broccoli	44.00
Lychees	45.00
Unsweetened apple juice	49.00
Orange	54.00
Kiwi fruit	59.00
Brussels sprouts	60.00
Strawberries	77.00
Blackcurrants	115.00

VITAMIN D
Micrograms per 100 g (3.5 oz)

Skimmed milk	0.01
Whole milk	0.03
Fromage frais	0.05
Cheddar cheese	0.26
Cornflakes	2.80
Rice Krispies	2.80
Kellogg's Start	4.20
Margarine	8.00

VITAMIN E
Milligrams per 100 g (3.5 oz)

Semi-skimmed milk	0.03
Boiled potatoes	0.06
Cucumber	0.07
Cottage cheese	0.08
Full-fat milk	0.09
Cabbage, boiled	0.10
Leg of lamb, cooked	0.10
Cauliflower	0.11
Roast chicken	0.11
Frozen peas	0.18
Red kidney beans, cooked	0.20
Wholemeal bread	0.20
Orange	0.24
Topside of beef, cooked	0.26
Banana	0.27
Brown rice, boiled	0.30
Grilled herring	0.30
Lamb's liver, fried	0.32
Baked beans	0.36
Cornflakes	0.40
Pear	0.50
Cheddar cheese	0.53
Carrots	0.56

Lettuce	0.57	Tomato	7.00
Cox's apple	0.59	White spaghetti, boiled	7.00
Grilled cod	0.59	Leg of lamb, cooked	8.00
Rice Krispies	0.60	Red peppers, raw	8.00
Plums	0.61	Roast chicken	9.00
Unsweetened orange juice	0.68	Roast turkey	9.00
Leeks	0.78	Avocado	11.00
Sweetcorn, boiled	0.88	Pear	11.00
Brussels sprouts	0.90	Butter	15.00
Broccoli	1.10	Cornflakes	15.00
Boiled egg	1.11	White rice, boiled	18.00
Tomato	1.22	Grilled cod	22.00
Watercress	1.46	Lentils, boiled	22.00
Parsley	1.70	Baked salmon	29.00
Spinach, boiled	1.71	Green peppers, raw	30.00
Olives	1.99	Young carrots	30.00
Butter	2.00	Grilled herring	33.00
Onions, dried raw	2.69	Wholemeal flour	38.00
Mushrooms, fried in corn oil	2.84	Turnips, baked	45.00
Avocado	3.20	Orange	47.00
Muesli	3.20	Baked beans	48.00
Walnuts	3.85	Wholemeal bread	54.00
Peanut butter	4.99	Boiled egg	57.00
Olive oil	5.10	Peanuts	60.00
Sweet potato, baked	5.96	Cottage cheese	73.00
Brazil nuts	7.18	Soya beans, boiled	83.00
Peanuts	10.09	White bread	100.00
Pine nuts	13.65	Full-fat milk	115.00
Rapeseed oil	18.40	Hovis	120.00
Almonds	23.96	Muesli	120.00
Hazelnuts	24.98	Skimmed milk	120.00
Sunflower oil	48.70	Semi-skimmed milk	120.00
		Prawns, boiled	150.00

CALCIUM
Milligrams per 100 g (3.5 oz)

		Spinach, boiled	150.00
		Brazil nuts	170.00
		Yoghurt, low-fat, plain	190.00
Cox's apple	4.00	Soya flour	210.00
Brown rice, boiled	4.00	Almonds	240.00
Potatoes, boiled	5.00	White self-raising flour	450.00
Banana	6.00	Sardines	550.00
Topside of beef, cooked	6.00	Sprats, fried	710.00
White pasta, boiled	7.00	Cheddar cheese	720.00

Whitebait, fried	860.00	Soya beans, boiled	3.00
		Lentils, boiled	3.50
IRON		Hovis	3.70
Milligrams per 100 g (3.5 oz)		Wholemeal flour	3.90
		Muesli	5.60
Semi-skimmed milk	0.05	Cornflakes	6.70
Skimmed milk	0.06	Rice Krispies	6.70
Full-fat milk	0.06	Soya flour	6.90
Cottage cheese	0.10		
Orange	0.10	**MAGNESIUM**	
Cox's apple	0.20	Milligrams per 100 g (3.5 oz)	
Pear	0.20		
White rice	0.20	Butter	2.00
Banana	0.30	Cox's apple	6.00
Cabbage, boiled	0.30	Turnip, baked	6.00
Cheddar cheese	0.30	Young carrots	6.00
Avocado	0.40	Tomato	7.00
Grilled cod	0.40	Cottage cheese	9.00
Potatoes, boiled	0.40	Orange	10.00
Young carrots, boiled	0.40	Full-fat milk	11.00
Brown rice, boiled	0.50	White rice, boiled	11.00
Tomato	0.50	Semi-skimmed milk	11.00
White pasta, boiled	0.50	Skimmed milk	12.00
Baked salmon	0.80	Boiled egg	12.00
Roast chicken	0.80	Cornflakes	14.00
Roast turkey	0.90	Potatoes, boiled	14.00
Grilled herring	1.00	Red peppers, raw	14.00
Red peppers, raw	1.00	White pasta	15.00
Boiled prawns	1.10	Wholemeal spaghetti, boiled	15.00
Green peppers, raw	1.20	White self-raising flour	20.00
Baked beans	1.40	Green peppers, raw	24.00
Wholemeal spaghetti, boiled	1.40	Roast chicken	24.00
White bread	1.60	Topside of beef, cooked	24.00
Spinach, boiled	1.70	White bread	24.00
Boiled egg	1.90	Avocado	25.00
White self-raising flour	2.00	Cheddar cheese	25.00
Brazil nuts	2.50	Grilled cod	26.00
Peanuts	2.50	Roast turkey	27.00
Leg of lamb, cooked	2.70	Leg of lamb, cooked	28.00
Wholemeal bread	2.70	Baked salmon	29.00
Topside of beef, cooked	2.80	Baked beans	31.00
Almonds	3.00	Spinach, boiled	31.00

Grilled herring	32.00	Pear	0.10
Banana	34.00	Orange	0.10
Lentils, boiled	34.00	Red peppers, raw	0.10
Boiled prawns	42.00	Banana	0.20
Wholemeal spaghetti, boiled	42.00	Young carrots	0.20
Brown rice, boiled	43.00	Cornflakes	0.30
Hovis	56.00	Potatoes, boiled	0.30
Soya beans, boiled	63.00	Avocado	0.40
Wholemeal bread	76.00	Full-fat milk	0.40
Muesli	85.00	Skimmed milk	0.40
Wholemeal flour	120.00	Green peppers, raw	0.40
Peanuts	210.00	Semi-skimmed milk	0.40
Soya flour	240.00	Baked beans	0.50
Almonds	270.00	Grilled cod	0.50
Brazil nuts	410.00	Grilled herring	0.50
		White pasta	0.50
		Tomatoes	0.50

SELENIUM
Micrograms per 100 g (3.5 oz)

		Cottage cheese	0.60
		Spinach, boiled	0.60
Full-fat milk	1.00	White bread	0.60
Semi-skimmed milk	1.00	White self-raising flour	0.60
Skimmed milk	1.00	Brown rice	0.70
Baked beans	2.00	White rice	0.70
Cornflakes	2.00	Soya beans, boiled	0.90
Orange	2.00	Wholemeal spaghetti, boiled	1.10
Peanuts	3.00	Boiled egg	1.30
Almonds	4.00	Lentils, boiled	1.40
Cottage cheese	4.00	Roast chicken	1.50
White rice	4.00	Boiled prawns	1.60
White self-raising flour	4.00	Wholemeal bread	1.80
Soya beans, boiled	5.00	Hovis	2.10
Boiled egg	11.00	Cheddar cheese	2.30
Cheddar cheese	12.00	Roast turkey	2.40
White bread	28.00	Muesli	2.50
Wholemeal bread	35.00	Wholemeal flour	2.90
Lentils, boiled	40.00	Almonds	3.20
Wholemeal flour	53.00	Peanuts	3.50
		Brazil nuts	4.20

ZINC
Milligrams per 100 g (3.5 oz)

		Leg of lamb, cooked	5.30
		Topside of beef, cooked	5.50
Butter	0.10		

ESSENTIAL FATTY ACIDS

Exact amounts of these fats are hard to quantify. Good sources for the two families of essential fatty acids are given.

OMEGA 6 SERIES ESSENTIAL
FATTY ACIDS

Sunflower oil
Rape seed oil
Corn oil
Almonds

Walnuts
Brazil nuts
Sunflower seeds
Soya products including Tofu

OMEGA 3 SERIES ESSENTIAL
FATTY ACIDS

Mackerel } fresh cooked or
Herring } smoked/pickled
Salmon }
Walnuts and walnut oil
Rape seed oil
Soya products and soy bean oil

Foods containing polyunsaturated fats

Certain fish contain essential oils, similar to those found in vegetables. These oils are helpful in maintaining skin quality and may also be of value in preventing pre-menstrual breast tenderness.

Herring
Mackerel
Pilchard
Salmon
Sardines
Sprats
Whitebait

HOW TO BEGIN

In the next chapter 'A tailor-made nutritional programme' you will find details about charting your symptoms and keeping daily diaries as a record of your progress. I suggest you do the following:

- Complete a chart before you begin so that you have a clear picture of your symptoms.
- Follow the specialized diet for a period of three months.
- Keep daily diaries of all your symptoms. These are provided on page 281 at the end of the book.
- Complete another chart after three months. This can then be compared with your first chart to measure your progress.

16

A TAILOR-MADE
NUTRITIONAL
PROGRAMME – OPTION 3

The tailor-made nutritional programme is designed to help overcome severe symptoms. Having said that, I feel I should also point out that it is a tough programme, and if your symptoms are extremely severe, you may need help initially. If you can't manage to work out your own programme or you feel you need support, you can contact us at the Women's Nutritional Advisory Service.

Before getting too enthusiastic, it's important to understand that 'The Nutritional Programme' involves quite a bit of work. It's not a magic pill or potion that works overnight in your sleep, but an organized regime that requires a substantial amount of will-power to start with.

At the Women's Nutritional Advisory Service we try to work out the best programme for each individual, according to their symptoms and their existing lifestyle. A *realistic* regime stands a good chance of being followed, whereas an idealistic programme that would work wonders in theory is useless if left in a drawer and forgotten about because it's just too difficult to face or follow.

In order to work out each individual's programme, we need a fair amount of information. As I don't have your chart in front of me I can't work out your programme in the usual way. What I *can* do is to set you a series of questions, and then explain to you, according to your answers, how you go about working out your own programme. I will be unveiling some 'trade secrets' in the course of this section of the book, and hopefully most aspects of the Pre-Menstrual Syndrome will have been covered.

YOUR PERSONAL NUTRITIONAL PROGRAMME

This programme is designed to help moderate and severe sufferers over their symptoms. If you feel your symptoms fit into the definition of moderate or severe on page 166, you would be best advised to follow this more specialized tailor-made nutritional plan. Make a start in completing the chart and the diary provided on pages 168 and 282. Once you are satisfied with your answers, usually after one full cycle, you can begin compiling your own programme.

If you prefer to begin immediately without waiting for the forms to be completed, then I suggest you follow Option 2 – A Specialized Dietary Plan on page 149. Once your precise programme has been formulated you can implement the additional recommendations and make any changes that are needed.

To avoid confusion, remember that recommendations according to your symptoms should be followed in the long term for best results, rather than continuing to follow the general recommendations made in previous chapters. The reason I make this point is that you may find the two sets of instructions conflict in some areas. An example is that the general recommendations suggest eating plenty of whole grains. However we often find that severe symptoms may be aggravated by certain grains and we may therefore suggest that these are omitted from the diet for a specific period of time in some cases. I have covered this in much fuller detail in the section on food allergies on page 179.

A STEP-BY-STEP GUIDE
TO WORK OUT YOUR OWN PROGRAMME

STEP ONE – HOW TO CHART YOUR SYMPTOMS

Begin by completing the first Pre-Menstrual Syndrome Chart on page 168. This should ideally be completed in two parts.

The left-hand column deals with how you feel normally when you are not pre-menstrual. *This column should be completed three days after your period has started or when you feel at your best.*

The right-hand column deals with how you feel pre-menstrually when your symptoms are at their worst. *This column should be completed two days before your period is due or when you feel at your worst.*

In order to work out your score, you must place a tick by each symptom in both columns. On page 167 is an example of a completed chart. You can see how the symptoms become far more severe pre-menstrually (on the right-hand side of the chart).

Severity of symptoms

You will notice that on the chart you are asked to assess whether your symptoms are mild, moderate or severe. Each of these categories has a numerical score as follows:

0 = None.
1 = Mild.
2 = Moderate.
3 = Severe.

Mild, moderate and severe defined

(1) Mild — Means that symptoms are present but they do not interfere with your activities. You feel all right, but are aware that some physical and emotional changes are taking place as your period approaches.

(2) Moderate — Means that symptoms are present and they do interfere with some activities, but they are not disabling. You feel well below par and maybe even cancel arrangements. The family would be aware your period is on its way, maybe even before you are.

(3) Severe — Means that symptoms are not only present, they interfere with all activities. They are severely disabling and it's likely that life would be pretty hard to cope with until the symptoms pass.

Using Anita's first chart on page 167 as an example, let's go through it section by section so that you can understand how it works.

PMS A, H, C and D

PMS A – Anxiety. In order to 'qualify' for PMS A your score must be 4 or above for this section. To get your final score you subtract the score for the week after your period from the score for the week before your period.

ANITA WALKER

SYMPTOMS

	WEEK AFTER PERIOD (Fill in 3 days after period)				WEEK BEFORE PERIOD (Fill in 2-3 days before period)			
	None	Mild	Moderate	Severe	None	Mild	Moderate	Severe
PMS - A								
Nervous Tension	✓							✓
Mood Swings	✓							✓
Irritability	✓							✓
Anxiety	✓							✓
PMS - H								
*Weight Gain	✓							✓
Swelling of Extremities			✓					✓
Breast Tenderness	✓							✓
Abdominal Bloating		✓						✓
PMS - C								
Headache	✓						✓	
Craving for Sweets	✓							✓
Increased Appetite	✓							✓
Heart Pounding	✓				✓			
Fatigue	✓							✓
Dizziness or Fainting	✓				✓			
PMS - D								
Depression	✓							✓
Forgetfulness	✓							✓
Crying	✓						✓	
Confusion	✓							✓
Insomnia	✓							✓
OTHER SYMPTOMS								
Loss of Sexual Interest	✓					✓		
Disorientation	✓							✓
Clumsiness	✓							✓
Tremors/Shakes	✓							✓
Thoughts of Suicide	✓							✓
Agoraphobia	✓							
Increased Physical Activity	✓				✓			
Heavy/Aching Legs	✓							✓
Generalized Aches	✓							✓
Bad Breath	✓							✓
Sensitivity to Music/Light	✓				✓			
Excessive Thirst	✓							✓

Do you have any other PRE-MENSTRUAL SYMPTOMS not listed above?

1. Argue with husband then contemplate leaving him and breaking

2. up the marriage – how we'd do it, finances etc.

3. Sensitivity to noise/find childrens questions and demands

4. unbearably intrusive.

*5. How much weight do you gain before your period?   7-10 lbs

SYMPTOMS

	WEEK AFTER PERIOD (Fill in 3 days after period)				WEEK BEFORE PERIOD (Fill in 2-3 days before period)			
	None	Mild	Moderate	Severe	None	Mild	Moderate	Severe
PMS - A								
Nervous Tension								
Mood Swings								
Irritability								
Anxiety								
PMS - H								
*Weight Gain								
Swelling of Extremities								
Breast Tenderness								
Abdominal Bloating								
PMS - C								
Headache								
Craving for Sweets								
Increased Appetite								
Heart Pounding								
Fatigue								
Dizziness or Fainting								
PMS - D								
Depression								
Forgetfulness								
Crying								
Confusion								
Insomnia								
OTHER SYMPTOMS								
Loss of Sexual Interest								
Disorientation								
Clumsiness								
Tremors/Shakes								
Thoughts of Suicide								
Agoraphobia								
Increased Physical Activity								
Heavy/Aching Legs								
Generalized Aches								
Bad Breath								
Sensitivity to Music/Light								
Excessive Thirst								

Do you have any other PRE-MENSTRUAL SYMPTOMS not listed above?

1. _____

2. _____

3. _____

4. _____

*5.　　How much weight do you gain before your period? _____

Anita scored 0 after her period and 12 pre-menstrually. Therefore, her overall score is 12, so she certainly does qualify for PMS A.

The reason for subtracting one score from another in this fashion is to attempt to get the *actual* pre-menstrual score. For example, if you have moderate regular headaches all month and they become severe pre-menstrually your real pre-menstrual headache score is only 1, as this symptom only moved from mild to moderate. Compare this to another person who usually has no headaches, but has severe pre-menstrual headaches: the pre-menstrual headache score would be 3 here.

Not to subtract the usual situation for the rest of your cycle from the pre-menstrual situation would create a false picture.

This method of scoring applies to all four categories.

PMS H – Hydration. For PMS H you also need a score of 4 to qualify. Anita scored 3 after her period and 10 before her period, giving her a total score of 7. She therefore qualifies.

PMS C – Sugar craving. For PMS C there are six symptoms. You will need an overall score of 6 to qualify. Anita scored 0 after her period and a score of 11 before her period. Her overall score was therefore 11.

PMS D – Depression. And finally for PMS D, a score of 5 is necessary as there are five symptoms listed in this category. Anita scored 0 after her period and 14 pre-menstrually. Her total score here was 14. She qualified with honours!

Once you have completed your chart you can go on to work out your scores using this example.

Each category has been dealt with separately. You may find that only one of the four categories applies to you. However, it is perfectly possible to be suffering from several categories, or in fact all four.

Now fill in your first chart and see how you fare.

You will notice an additional section on the chart. This is made up of other symptoms which have been reported repeatedly by patients.

Is it really pre-menstrual?

The best way to assess your symptoms in order to confirm that they are pre-menstrual is to keep daily diaries as I mentioned previously. After two or three months you will see a definite pattern emerging which will serve to confirm the diagnosis of PMS. Two diaries have been provided for this purpose beginning on page 283. Please feel free to photocopy the diaries if you wish.

If, after three months, it seems that your scores are low and your symptoms seem to be persisting all month rather than pre-menstrually, then it would be best to have a full medical consultation and physical examination to determine whether there is some other problem.

Diaries

It is not only a good idea, but essential that you keep daily diaries. In fact, some doctors feel that it is necessary to keep a diary for three months in order to confirm the diagnosis of PMS. There are several reasons for this:

- To keep a check on your symptoms.

- To confirm that you have PMS.

- To show a pattern of when the symptoms occur each month.

- To have as a record so that you can judge whether improvement is occurring, without having to rely on your memory.

The form we use is called the Menstrual Symptomatology Diary (MSD). It was designed by Dr Abraham originally and was subsequently expanded by us. It enables sufferers to keep an ongoing record of their symptoms. The diary should be filled in at the end of each day, throughout the cycle. There are a few things to remember when you do this:

The first day of your cycle is the day your period begins. Whether your period comes every 22 days or 32 days is irrelevant here. The day bleeding begins, you start a new diary calling this *Day 1*.

There is an example of a completed diary opposite.

Now you should start filling in the diary and continue to fill it in at the end of each day.

After a few months you should see a very definite pattern emerging. The most likely pattern is for you to experience few symptoms once your period has arrived until at least ovulation, that is, mid-cycle. So you will fill in only noughts in the diary. If you have any symptoms at ovulation, indicate them vertically, according to their severity. As your period approaches, the number you fill in will probably get higher, at least for the symptoms that bother you.

MENSTRUAL SYMPTOMATOLOGY DIARY

Name: _____

GRADING OF MENSES

0–none	3–heavy
1–slight	4–heavy and
2–moderate	clots

GRADING OF SYMPTOMS (COMPLAINTS)

0–none
1–mild-present but does not interfere with activities
2–moderate-present and interferes with activities but not disabling
3–severe-disabling. Unable to function.

Day of cycle	1	2	3	4	5	6	7	8	9	10	11	12	13	14	15	16	17	18	19	20	21	22	23	24	25	26	27	28	29
Date	13	14	15	16	17	18	19	20	21	22	23	24	25	26	27	28	29	30	31	1	2	3	4	5	6	7	8	9	10
Period	1	2	3	3	2	1	0	0	0	0	0	0	0	0	0	0	0	0	0	0	0	0	0	0	0	0	0	0	0

PMS - A

	1	2	3	4	5	6	7	8	9	10	11	12	13	14	15	16	17	18	19	20	21	22	23	24	25	26	27	28	29
Nervous tension	1	0	0	0	0	0	0	0	0	0	0	0	0	0	0	0	0	0	1	0	1	1	2	2	3	3	3	3	2
Mood swings	0	0	0	0	0	0	0	0	0	0	0	0	0	0	0	0	0	1	2	1	2	2	3	2	3	2	2	2	3
Irritability	0	0	0	0	0	0	0	0	0	0	0	0	0	0	0	0	0	0	0	1	1	2	2	2	2	2	3	3	3
Anxiety	0	0	0	0	0	0	0	0	0	0	0	0	0	0	0	0	1	1	0	0	2	3	3	2	2	2	3	2	

PMS - H

	1	2	3	4	5	6	7	8	9	10	11	12	13	14	15	16	17	18	19	20	21	22	23	24	25	26	27	28	29
Weight gain	0	0	0	0	0	0	0	0	0	0	0	0	0	0	0	0	0	0	1	1	1	1	2	2	2	3	2	3	3
Swelling of extremities	0	0	0	0	0	0	0	0	0	0	0	0	0	0	0	0	0	0	0	0	1	1	1	1	2	2	2	2	2
Breast tenderness	0	0	0	0	0	0	0	0	0	0	0	0	0	0	0	0	0	0	0	1	1	1	1	2	2	2	2	2	2
Abdominal bloating	1	0	0	0	0	0	0	0	0	0	0	0	0	0	0	0	0	1	1	2	2	2	1	2	1	1	2	2	2

PMS - C

	1	2	3	4	5	6	7	8	9	10	11	12	13	14	15	16	17	18	19	20	21	22	23	24	25	26	27	28	29
Headache	0	0	0	1	0	0	0	0	0	0	0	0	0	0	0	0	0	0	0	0	0	0	0	0	2	0	0	0	1
Craving for sweets	0	0	0	0	0	0	0	0	0	0	0	0	0	0	0	1	2	2	0	1	2	3	3	3	2	1	2	2	2
Increased appetite	0	0	0	0	0	0	0	0	0	0	0	0	0	0	0	0	3	2	2	1	0	0	2	2	2	2	2	2	2
Heart pounding	0	0	0	0	0	0	0	0	0	0	0	0	0	0	0	0	0	0	0	0	0	0	0	0	0	0	0	0	0
Fatigue	1	1	2	1	0	0	0	0	0	0	0	0	0	0	0	0	0	0	0	0	2	2	3	3	3	3	3	3	3
Dizziness or faintness	1	0	0	0	0	0	0	0	0	0	0	0	0	0	0	0	0	0	0	0	0	0	0	0	0	0	0	0	0

PMS - D

	1	2	3	4	5	6	7	8	9	10	11	12	13	14	15	16	17	18	19	20	21	22	23	24	25	26	27	28	29
Depression	1	0	0	1	0	0	0	0	0	0	0	0	0	0	0	0	0	0	1	1	1	2	2	2	3	3	3	3	3
Forgetfulness	0	0	0	0	0	0	0	0	0	0	0	0	0	0	0	0	1	0	3	2	3	3	3	3	3	3	2	2	3
Crying	0	0	0	0	0	0	0	0	0	0	0	0	0	0	0	0	1	0	1	2	1	2	3	3	3	3	2	3	3
Confusion	1	0	0	0	0	0	0	0	0	0	0	0	0	0	0	0	0	1	2	2	2	2	2	3	3	2	2	2	2
Insomnia	1	1	0	0	0	0	0	0	0	0	0	0	0	0	0	0	0	1	1	1	1	1	2	2	2	1	3	3	3

PAIN

	1	2	3	4	5	6	7	8	9	10	11	12	13	14	15	16	17	18	19	20	21	22	23	24	25	26	27	28	29
Cramps (low abdominal)																													
Backache																													
General aches/pains																													
Frequency of sex (tick day)																													
Enjoyment of sex (0-10)																													

NOTES:

STEP TWO – PLANNING YOUR DIET

Making changes

Unfortunately there seems to be some truth in the saying 'old habits die hard'. If you set out bearing this in mind you won't get disillusioned along the way. Following the programme usually involves making quite a few changes in both diet and lifestyle. To be realistic, it does take a while to adjust fully. The first month is usually the most rocky. The new routine may cause a bit of confusion here and there at first and a few surprises along the way. If it seems difficult, remember, it is important to persist until you are out of the woods.

Forewarned is forearmed

Withdrawal symptoms may occur during the first few days on the programme, and can sometimes last for as long as one or two weeks if you are unfortunate. Whilst you shouldn't definitely expect these, it's worth bearing in mind that they are very common. Depriving the body of things which it has grown used to sometimes causes it to 'bite back'. It may seem a strange concept that this should occur as a result of dietary changes. However, it is fairly similar to the mechanism of withdrawing from drugs or alcohol. Due to the possible withdrawal symptoms from certain foods and drinks, it is better not to begin this diet in your pre-menstrual phase. Make a start after your period has arrived.

Giving up tea and coffee, for example, may trigger off a number of changes in the body. These may cause you to feel tired or uptight, anxious and on edge. Headaches may occur and, more often, the desire to eat seems to persist. You will be pleased to hear that all this tends to settle down within days, certainly within a couple of weeks. Once you have passed this stage, if it happens to you at all, life becomes much easier, and before long you will notice new habit patterns forming. So much so that patients often prefer *not* to return to their former habits, simply because their tastes have changed! For example, they lose their desire for salty food and regular cups of strong coffee.

The general consensus of opinion is that it is worth persevering, for there is a light at the end of the tunnel. Our research proves this conclusively. When the Women's Nutritional Advisory Service had been in existence for one year we decided it would be desirable to get some scientific feedback on our results. We looked at the results of a group of women who had been on the programme. They had made dietary changes, taken nutritional supplements and regularly exercised. After three months

172

89 per cent of the women reported that they felt significantly better and there was a 91 per cent reduction in severe symptoms.

We are also reminded that our efforts are worthwhile by the constant flow of grateful letters we receive from patients and their partners. From reading the case histories in Part One you will have had a taste of the magnitude of the original problems and then read about incredible changes that took place. The letters we receive from women who have completed the programme often read like fairy stories. It is no wonder we are keen to see the natural approach to curing PMS being widely used!

If I haven't put you off – let's get down to it! We'll deal with dietary aspects first of all, then supplement recommendations..

First of all, decide from your chart which are your main pre-menstrual symptoms. Refer to the section 'PMS and Other Related Symptoms' on page 149 and decide which vitamins and minerals you should be concentrating on in particular. Then read through the food lists starting on page 155 to familiarize yourself with the foods high in the relevant nutrient. If you are suffering severely, it's likely to encompass most of the food groups.

LET'S PUT YOU UNDER THE MICROSCOPE

Some of your symptoms fall into categories which you have now been able to identify, but for severe PMS sufferers there are often other factors which play a major part in their condition. In order to determine whether any of these factors apply to you personally, you will need to examine several groups of symptoms. I have put certain symptoms into groups to make this simpler.

On the next page there is a skeleton chart for you to complete as you go along. As you read through the sections that follow, make a note of each recommendation which you feel applies to you. By the time you have finished reading the whole of Part Three of this book you should have your programme noted down for easy reference. A copy of this can be pinned up in your kitchen to remind you of the Dos and Don'ts.

PERSONAL NUTRITIONAL PROGRAMME
SUMMARY OF RECOMMENDATIONS

Diet section

1.

2.

3.

4.

5.

6.

7.

8.

9.

10.

Supplement section

1.

2.

3.

4.

5.

GENERAL RECOMMENDATIONS

There are general recommendations that should be implemented by all severe sufferers, almost regardless of which categories of PMS they suffer from. The fact that you need to cut out certain food groups now does not mean this will remain so for ever. It is simply a way of giving your body a rest and allowing it to recover. I will explain later how to go about re-introducing some of the foods into your diet.

1. Cut out caffeine

Caffeine is addictive, although we do not readily believe it to be so. It is present in tea, coffee, chocolate and cola-based drinks.

Caffeine and some other similar substances tend to aggravate PMS A symptoms, i.e. anxiety, irritability, mood swings and nervous tension. It also affects breast symptoms, and the PMS D symptoms of depression and insomnia.

It is advisable to cut caffeine out completely, and to consume only small amounts of decaffeinated coffee, as this contains other chemicals which may have an effect on PMS symptoms. Fortunately, there are many pleasant alternatives which you will find in healthfood shops.

- There are many varieties of herb tea, some fruity and some more herby in taste, most of which are caffeine-free. The most 'tea-like' substitute we have found is 'Redbush' or 'Rooibosch' tea. This can be made with or without milk. Many former tea addicts have found that after a week or two it tastes far more pleasant than ordinary tea. You will need to shop around and experiment to find teas that suit your palate.

- Dandelion coffee is certainly worth a try. It comes in instant form and in roasted root form. I like to use the root, which I put through my coffee filter.

- There are numerous other cereal alternatives you could try, all of which you should find in a good healthfood shop.

2. Keep your dairy consumption moderate

Aim to consume two servings of dairy products per day as well as milk in your drinks, if required. This means you can have milk and yoghurt with cereals and one other serving of yoghurt or cheese each day. Refer to the list of calcium rich foods on p. 160 and make sure you consume calcium from non-dairy sources. Eating a calcium-rich diet can help to prevent osteoporosis, the bone thinning disease.

3. Keep your salt intake to a minimum

Salt may play a part in Pre-Menstrual Syndrome. Either in the cooking or added at the table, salt leads to increased water retention which tends to aggravate many of the PMS symptoms. You should also avoid eating salty foods. A diet low in salt is a good idea for many reasons, as well as being of value in the treatment of some of your symptoms. If you have an irresistible desire for salt, try using a salt substitute such as LoSalt which is rich in potassium salt, rather than the commonly available sodium salt. You will find that after you have been avoiding salt for three or four weeks you no longer miss it, and will begin to taste the food itself.

4. Keep your sugar intake low

Refined sugar contains no vitamins or minerals but does require good nutrients in order to be metabolized. Foods that have a high sugar content, such as cakes, biscuits (cookies) chocolate, jam (jelly), some puddings, soft drinks and ice cream are high in calories, but have a low nutrient content. Sugar and sweet foods such as cakes, biscuits, cookies, puddings, jam (jelly), soft drinks and ice cream are high in calories (kjs) and low in important vitamins and minerals. It is deficiencies in some of these vitamins and minerals which play such a part in pre-menstrual symptoms, particularly vitamin B6 and magnesium. Having a lot of sugar in your diet may also contribute significantly to fluid retention and therefore should be avoided.

It is not widely appreciated that 'junk food' contains a lot of phosphorus, which is known to block the uptake of certain trace minerals. Without these important trace minerals PMS symptoms tend to get worse. By 'junk food' we mean processed food, refined food, prepared food, i.e. packet soups, cakes, etc. and anything that contains added sugar, such as sweets (candy), cakes, biscuits (cookies), chocolates and soft drinks.

This is not a no-sugar diet, but certainly low sugar. Reducing your sugar intake, especially if you have been a large consumer, can be difficult initially, but there are a number of acceptable alternatives.

- Low-sugar or sugar-free fruit juice and nut bars can be found in many healthfood shops and used in place of sweets.

- Concentrated apple juice is a good sweetener when cooking. Small amounts of molasses may also be used as it is high in the B vitamins and magnesium.

- There are sugar-free jams (jellies) available in healthfood shops. These are made with fruit and apple juice.

- Watered-down fruit juice is a good substitute for soft drinks as it contains no extra sugar or colouring agents etc.

- Sweeteners can be used in drinks.

Unfortunately, honey consists mainly of sugar, and only one or two teaspoons should be consumed a day if you can't resist it. Similarly, small amounts of refined sugar – one teaspoon per day – may also be allowed.

The same goes for brown sugar, as it has more or less the same effect on your metabolism.

There are specific supplement recommendations for sugar cravings which are mentioned on pages 198 and 205.

5. Limit your intake of alcohol

As I mentioned in Chapter 11, regular alcohol consumption can have devastating consequences on the body. Alcohol is known to block absorption of certain trace minerals and to knock out B vitamins from the system. Without these you are far more prone to pre-menstrual symptoms. Try not to consume more than two or three alcoholic drinks per week. Fortunately, there are now alcohol-free wines and beers on the market, so you need not refuse a drink.

6. Reduce cigarette smoking

Smoking may affect the levels of certain vitamins, particularly vitamin C, and also aggravate pre-menstrual breast tenderness as well as PMS A symptoms. It is advisable, therefore, that your cigarette consumption be substantially reduced. You may find it easier to cut down on smoking once you have been on the programme for a few weeks. If you don't succeed at first, try again after a month. One sneaky way to cut down gradually without noticing too much is to wait five or ten minutes before lighting up each time so that the distance between cigarettes slowly becomes greater.

7. Eat your greens!

Green leafy vegetables are the major source of some important vitamins and in particular contain the mineral magnesium which plays a substantial part in the correction of pre-menstrual symptoms. It is vital, therefore, that you have a good helping of salad or green leafy vegetables every day. The greens should preferably be lightly cooked in the minimum of water to preserve their vitamin and mineral content. By careful attention to your diet in the long term, your need for vitamin and mineral supplements should be reduced once your symptoms are under control.

8. Eat plenty of raw food

Uncooked food is usually far more nutritious than food that has been cooked. In most cooking processes as much as half of the nutrients are lost.

Raw food has a much higher fibre content, too. Aim to eat at least one, and preferably two raw meals per day. Eat plenty of salad stuff, fruit and raw vegetables, all of which are easy to prepare and fairly portable, if you are eating away from home. An excellent book to refer to is *The New Raw Energy* by Leslie and Susannah Kenton which is mentioned on the Recommended Reading List on page 274.

9. A note to vegetarians and vegans

Vegetarians who do not eat meat or fish, and vegans who only consume vegetable produce may need to pay particular attention to certain aspects of their diet, so that they do not become nutritionally deficient. Whilst there are many vegetarians who take great care over their diets, there are still too many who try to exist on lettuce leaves and the like. Apart from all the recommendations made so far, vegetarians and vegans should concentrate on the following:

- Make sure you have an adequate balance of proteins in your diet.

- No single vegetarian protein contains all the appropriate nutrients required, so it's important to combine the different types of vegetable proteins in your vegetarian meals. Vegetarian proteins include: nuts, seeds, peas, beans, lentils, whole grains, brown rice, sprouted beans and soya bean products.

- Whilst beans are particularly nutritious, they often cause abdominal wind. Soaking them for 24 hours before cooking them and de-husking them may reduce the problem.

10. Iron and Zinc

Ensure you have an adequate intake of the minerals iron and zinc. You can check on this by referring to the iron and zinc food lists which can be found on pages 161–162.

MORE SPECIALIZED PROBLEMS: SECTIONS 1–8

I have split this section up into symptom groups. After reading through the group of symptoms, there are recommendations. If these symptoms apply to you, make a note of the recommendation on your personal chart. If the symptoms don't apply to you, then simply pass on to the next section.

Do you suffer with any of the following? (tick applicable boxes)

Abdominal bloating	☐	Depression	☐
Excessive wind	☐	Mouth ulcers	☐
Constipation	☐	Fatigue	☐
Diarrhoea	☐		

If you ticked any two of these symptoms it would be *desirable* for you to follow the following recommendations.

If, however, you ticked three or more it is *advisable* for you to read through the recommendations carefully, mark them on your chart, and apply them.

SECTION 1: SENSITIVITY TO GRAINS

There is evidence to show that the symptoms mentioned in sections 1 to 8 may be related to food sensitivity. Research suggests that a significant percentage of the population produce antibodies to some foods. In our experience, this may be only a temporary state of affairs that occurs when we are not in very good nutritional shape when the immune system may be improved. Finding the right kind of diet for your body will help to overcome your symptoms. It is therefore worth avoiding certain groups of foods temporarily if you suffer with the symptoms in this section. Try to follow the recommendations closely – you will reap the benefit.

WHOLEWHEAT AND GRAINS: ALTERNATIVES

Many symptoms such as irritability, abdominal bloating, constipation, diarrhoea, excessive wind, irritable bowel, fatigue and depression can be aggravated by eating foods containing wheat and other grains. Certain people react to wheat, oats, barley and rye, and all foods made from them or containing them. They are therefore better off avoiding them altogether initially, until the symptoms are under control. It sounds a bit drastic, but there are lots of alternative foods that can be used instead, so don't despair.

Bread

There are now many alternatives to ordinary bread, some of which can be purchased and others which you need to bake yourself. Both chemists and healthfood shops usually have some stocks of the alternative grain products; in our experience the chemists are usually the most reasonably priced. Behind the counter in the pharmacy you will usually find a stock of products kept for people with gluten allergy. Ask the pharmacist for help, as they sometimes have to order products in on request.

Look out for some of the following products:

- Ener G white or brown rice bread (which toasts nicely)

- Glutafin wheat-free bread and rolls

- Rice cakes

- Glutano makes a flat bread like pumpernickel called 'Wholewheat' which is made from rice and corn. It is lovely as a base for open sandwiches.

- There are a number of very acceptable crackers these days. Glutano crackers are my favourite but Orgran and Glutafin make rice-corn and rice crackers, all of which are available from healthfood shops. Rice cakes, which are now available as squares, are also widely available in healthfood shops and supermarkets. It is worth noting that pharmacists can usually order wheat-free products such as Glutano crackers and Ener G rice bread at a slightly lower price than healthfood shops.

Home-made bread. Whilst I have not been very successful in making bread with alternative flours, some of our patients have successfully experimented. Look out for the recipes for potato and rice bread, and buckwheat and rice bread, on page 225.

Pasta

Although you will need to avoid the pasta made with wheat, there are many reasonable alternatives you can try. Most of these are available from healthfood shops, the Chinese supermarket or the pharmacist.

- **Pastariso** make brown rice spaghetti, which is very acceptable slightly undercooked. They also do a range of other pastas. Although some healthfood shops do stock it, it is easier to order it from the chemist.

- **Orgran** do a range of pasta made from alternative grains which is very popular with our patients.

- **Glutafin** have a range of pasta which is sometimes available in healthfood shops, and again can be ordered from the chemist.

- **Rice noodles** are available in a wide variety from Chinese supermarkets. There are wide flat rice noodles that resemble tagliatelli, spaghetti-like noodles, and the very skinny variety that only need soaking in a covered pan in boiling water for a few minutes. You will probably find that these are cheaper than the alternative pastas available from healthfood shops and chemists.

Breakfast cereal

Any rice or corn cereals will be fine, even the ordinary Rice Krispies and Cornflakes from the supermarkets. Add some chopped fruit and some crumbled nuts, perhaps a few seeds and a little dried fruit to your cereal to make it a bit more wholesome or try the recipe for alternative muesli on page 209. There are some alternative mueslis available in the shops, but they are usually very expensive for only a small packet.

Home-made cakes

If you enjoy cooking there are plenty of very acceptable biscuits, cakes, pastries, sponges and pancakes you can make using alternative flours. If you have never used any of the alternative flours before it may take you a little time to find the consistency that you like.

Sponge Brown rice flour is probably the best for making sponge. Make it up to the weight given in the recipe by mixing it with a little ground almond and a raising agent (cream of tartar and bicarbonate of soda).

Raising agents As baking powder contains wheat, you will need to use an alternative. Either use a combination of one part of bicarbonate of soda to two parts of cream of tartar, or use Glutafin wheat-free baking powder.

Savoury pancakes These can be made with pure buckwheat flour, which is part of the rhubarb family and tends to be quite heavy, or buckwheat mixed with a little white rice flour, which is very light.

Sweet pancakes are best made with a combination of brown rice flour, or ground rice, and cornflour, purchased form a healthfood shop or Chinese supermarket. Use half cornflour and half rice flour to replace the normal quantity of flour in the ordinary pancake recipe.

Breadcrumbs or batter A crisp coating for fish or meat can be made with maize meal, which can be found in the healthfood shop. Coat the fish or meat with maize meal, then with beaten egg, and once again with maize meal. You can then bake, grill or even fry the food which should emerge with a crispy coat.

Biscuits There are varieties of biscuits that you can make using brown rice flour, or ground rice, and ground nuts or coconut. If you make plain biscuits you can flavour them with lemon or ginger. Our recipes for almond macaroons and coconut biscuits are very acceptable, and at the same time more nutritious than the average biscuit as they are full of eggs and nuts. It's an idea to make some and keep them in the freezer so that you can take a few out when you really feel you need something sweet to eat.

There are many other flours that you can use in your cooking. Gram flour made from chickpeas, potato flour, soya flour and tapioca flour, are all good examples, but they are expensive. Glutafin make flour mixes for bread, pastry and cakes, as do True Free, and these are available in some healthfood shops.

Shop-bought cakes and biscuits

Acceptable cakes and biscuits can now be purchased in healthfood shops and ordered from most chemists.

Glutafin have a range of biscuits including digestives, and Rite-Diet and Glutano have a range of biscuits and cakes. The coconut biscuits are the least sweet, and the banana or lemon cakes are worth trying too. Look out for 'Protein' biscuits in the health food shops made by Granny Ann. These are soya based and popular with patients.

Snacks

It's nice to have something to crunch on when you are avoiding wheat. There are lots of corn products available, but do remember to read the labels as some have added wheat in the form of modified starch. Try corn chips, crisps, and wafers, and look in the Mexican section of the supermarket. Also, poppadoms are fine, and little mini spiced poppadoms are nice to nibble on or dip.

ASSESSING FOR GRAIN SENSITIVITY

You will need to become a nutritional detective by doing the following:

- Stop eating all the grains mentioned earlier (wheat, oats, barley, rye) for at least a month, preferably six weeks. You can eat one slice of French bread per day if you are desperate! But it's better to try to manage on rice crackers or rice cakes instead. This may seem strange as refined bread is nowhere near as nutritious as wholemeal bread.

However, during the refining process most of the grain has been removed and therefore the degree of aggravation caused by this is far less than by a wholegrain loaf.

- After a month or six weeks, or longer, when you feel that your symptoms have diminished, try introducing the various grains one by one to your diet. Begin just after a period, so that you don't confuse any reaction with PMS symptoms. Choose one grain, e.g. rye in the form of rye crackers. Introduce this into your diet and eat this for several days. If you have no reaction after five days, choose another grain and repeat this process. *DO NOT MIX the grains initially* because if you do get a reaction you won't know exactly what you have reacted to! Continue to do this with all the grains, providing you don't have reactions to any one of them. Try wheat last as it is the most common grain to cause problems. Keep good notes of your symptoms while you are reintroducing grains.

Once you get used to using the alternatives you shouldn't find the diet difficult to stick to. If you are going to avoid eating certain groups of foods for any length of time, it is important to arm yourself with all the alternative foods you can muster. It is not a weight-loss diet (although you might find that you lose weight if you are overweight) so you can literally eat as much as you like of the foods on your list. Never allow yourself to get hungry and never miss a meal. It's important to keep up a steady flow of good nutrients in order to allow your hormone and brain chemical metabolism to function at an optimum.

What to do if you have a reaction

The reactions may include diarrhoea or constipation, excessive wind, abdominal bloating, headaches, weight gain, fatigue, confusion, depression, mouth ulcers, rash, irritability and palpitations.

1. Once you have established what you have reacted to, make a note of it and avoid eating this food at all for now. This doesn't mean that you won't be able to eat this food again ever, but it is best avoided for now.

2. Wait until things have settled down again and then try again with another grain.

I appreciate that cutting out all grains is a severe measure. I suggest you begin by just cutting out wholewheat products. You will need to do this for at least four to six weeks to see whether there is any improvement. You can remain on small amounts of white or French bread.

Constipation

If constipation is a particular problem you might like to try taking some linseed. You can find some very palatable forms of it at your healthfood shop such as Linusit Gold. It is pleasant to eat and can easily be included in your breakfast cereals or salad.

Foods containing grains

It's surprising how many foods contain grains. Before I began 'label reading' I would never have believed the extent to which grains are used. It's a good exercise to go around the supermarket, reading labels on packets to get an idea of this for yourself. Sometimes labels aren't as explicit as they might be and they just contain the words 'edible starch'. This has to be regarded with suspicion if you are on a grain-free diet. Labelling of food in healthfood shops is usually more reliable and precise.

Wheat The most obvious foods containing wheat are bread, biscuits, cakes and flour made from wheat etc., but wheat is often present in prepared sauces, soups, and processed foods in general. Gluten-free products are not particularly recommended on a wheat-free diet as some of them still contain wheat.

The following list will give you a rough idea of what to look out for, but I suggest you make a practice of reading labels thoroughly before buying anything.

- Bread, particularly wholemeal, wheatmeal, etc. as these contain more of the natural wheat.

- Cakes, biscuits, pasta, spaghetti, macaroni etc. – pastry, pies, buns, bran (except rice or soya bran), and many breakfast cereals and sausages.

Oats Porridge, oat cookies and oat flakes.
Rye Rye bread (which may also contain wheat), rye crackers and pumpernickel.
Barley Often found in packet/tinned soups and stews, barley beverages.
Corn Corn on the cob, corn starch, corn (maize), oil and popcorn.

There are many lovely recipe books available with further ideas listed in the Recommended Reading section on page 274.

I have prepared some sample menus to give you an idea of the scope possible. There are also a few recipes included in the recipe section on page 208 as a guideline.

GRAIN FREE ALLERGY DIET

SAMPLE DAILY MENU – WHEAT, OATS, BARLEY AND RYE FREE

Breakfast

Cornflakes or Rice Krispies with:
    a piece of chopped fruit (e.g. a banana, some grapes, berries etc.)
    a few crumbled pecan nuts
    a tablespoon of pine nuts
    a tablespoon of raisins (if not avoiding yeast)
with milk or yoghurt

Followed by:

One or two slices of alternative toast with low sugar jam or marmalade

Alternatively:

2 scrambled eggs or omelette with grilled tomatoes
or boiled or poached eggs
Alternative crackers and low sugar spreads

Mid-morning snack

See **Snack list** overleaf.

Lunch

Jacket potato with a nutritious filling, for example:
    Tuna and sweetcorn with a little sour cream and black pepper
    Prawns
    Baked beans
    Curried chicken

or

Cold meat or fresh or tinned fish with salad

or

Rice noodles, or alternative pasta, and vegetables

or

Home-made soup and salad

Tea-time snack

See **Snack list**.

Dinner

Poultry/fish/meat *or* vegetarian protein served with three portions of vegetables.

Fresh fruit *or* a fresh fruit salad, or choose an appropriate sweet from the dessert section in this book starting on page 222 or from the *Beat PMT Cookbook*.

Snack list

raw vegetables and dips like hummus, taramasalata or guacamole
fresh fruit, nuts or seeds
yoghurt and fruit
alternative crackers and spreads like Whole Earth peanut butter
or low sugar jam
corn chips
mini poppadoms
rice salad with fruit and nuts
dried fruit bars

Beverages

Coffee substitutes. Dandelion coffee, chicory, or up to two cups of decaffeinated coffee per day.

Herbal teas. Rooibosch Eleven O'clock tea (with milk). This herbal tea 'look alike', available from healthfood shops, contains a mild, natural muscle relaxant and may help alleviate tension and ease period pains. It is favoured by many of our patients and is definitely worth a try. Other suggestions are bramble, raspberry and ginseng, mixed berry, lemon verbena, fennel and wild strawberry. These days most healthfood shops sell single sachets so that you can 'buy and try' without being saddled with a whole box of tea bags that you absolutely detest.

Cold drinks. Bottled water with or without fruit juice, mineral water, Appletise, Citrus Spring or other spring water and fruit juice preparations.

B = Breakfast   L = Lunch   D = Dinner   S = Sweet

For recipes, see Chapter 17, page 208.

OPTION 3 – FAST OPTION LUNCHES

Have a salad with:
    Home-made soup (or supermarket equivalent without modified starch)
    Jacket potato with a filling such as cheese, beans, tuna, sweetcorn and margarine
    Turkey or chicken
    Sardines, mackerel or pilchards; wheat-free crackers
    Rice noodles and stir-fry vegetables
    Beans on wheat-free toast (see page 185 for alternatives to wheat and page 225 for recipe for bread)
    Glutano crackers or rice cakes with cheese
    Greek salad
    Rice salad with almonds
    Danish open sandwich on Glutano wholewheat bread (made from rice and corn)
    Fresh fruit, nuts and yoghurt
    Raw vegetable crudité woth humus, taramasalata or guacamole and corn wafers or poppadoms
    Cheese omelette
    Avocado and salsa

OPTION 3 – FAST OPTION DINNERS

Have three portions of vegetables, including a green leafy vegetable if appropriate
    Broccoli and cauliflower cheese with a jacket potato
    Fresh grilled sardines and salad
    Kangaroo steak and chips
    Stir-fry vegetables with chicken, nuts, beans or Quorn, with rice or rice noodles
    Poached salmon with new potatoes
    Grilled lamb chops
    Corn tacos with mince or beans, sour cream, guacamole and salsa with salad
    Spaghetti bolognaise with rice noodles or corn pasta
    Grilled mackerel and salad
    Corn pasta with tomato sauce, pine nuts and fresh herbs
    Prepared Quorn and sweet-corn escalopes (frozen)
    Hard-boiled egg and grated cheese salad
    Mixed bean salad with mixed salad

A SAMPLE MENU PLAN FOR ONE WEEK

DAY 1

B   Orange juice
Buckwheat pancakes (crêpes)
Dried fruit conserve
L   Fresh avocado and tomato
     soup
Jacket potato with cheese
D   Cold mackerel fillets or
     Prince's Mackerel in Spicy
     Tomato Sauce
Green salad
Brown rice salad
S   Baked stuffed apples

DAY 2

B   ½ grapefruit
Mushroom omelette
L   Sliced turkey
Orange and beanshoot salad
Banana
D   Stir-fry vegetables and brown
     rice
S   Grain-free carrot cake

DAY 3

B   Apple juice
Orange and apple salad with
     millet flakes and nuts
L   Stuffed tomatoes
Waldorf salad (using sunflower
     seeds and nuts)
D   Grilled trout
Green leafy vegetables
Carrots and parsnips in herb
     sauce (thickened with
     potato flour)
Boiled potatoes
S   Banana cream

DAY 4

B   ½ grapefruit
Hot fruit breakfast
L   Tuna omelette
Salad
D   Rosemary and garlic lamb
Brown rice
Jacket potato garnished with
     (bell) peppers and parsley
S   Slice of apple and cinnamon
     cake

DAY 5

B   Orange juice
Buckwheat pancakes (crêpes)
     with tomatoes, (bell) pepper
     and herbs
L   Leek soup
Jacket potato with prawns
     (shrimps)
Plums
D   Roast chicken
Leaf greens
Carrots
Sprouts and turnips
Boiled potatoes
S   Dried fruit compote and yoghurt

DAY 6

B   ½ grapefruit
Smoked haddock
Mushrooms, tomatoes
L   Green salad
Rice salad and dressing
Apple
D   Liver and onions
Green vegetables
Sauté potatoes
S   Fruity cakes

DAY 7

B   Cornflakes
     Banana, sliced
     Crumbled pecan nuts
     1 tbsp raisins
     Yoghurt or milk

L   Savoury buckwheat pancakes
     (crêpes) with salmon, tuna
     or mackerel filling

D   Colourful lentils and salad

S   Fruit jelly

Snacks

With attention focused very much on food, you may get the 'munchies' for a few weeks. There are a number of things to eat between meals which will prevent you from dipping into the cookie jar!

1. Rice crackers or rice cakes from the healthfood shop or Glutano crackers. The crackers are particularly nice spread with peanut butter, sesame spread or sugar-free jam (jelly), all these from healthfood shops, too.

2. Sunflower seeds or other seeds from healthfood shops are pleasant to nibble between meals.

3. Unsalted nuts can be eaten freely, but limit intake of peanuts, which are somewhat indigestible.

4. Fresh fruit of your choice.

5. Rice biscuits or sesame biscuits and healthfood bars that don't contain wheat. Watch out for the sugar, though!

6. Dried fruit – preferably organic – which is both intrinsically sweet and rich in magnesium.

SECTION 2: SENSITIVITY TO YEAST

Do you suffer from any of the following symptoms?

Thrush (more than two episodes in the last five years) ☐

Itchy bottom ☐

Bloated abdomen ☐

Cracking at the corners of your mouth ☐

Depression ☐

Excessive wind ☐

Cystitis ☐

Two or more episodes of thrush and/or any other two symptoms certainly qualify you for the yeast-free diet.

YEAST SENSITIVITY

Yeast problems in the gut are very common it seems, and they can produce or aggravate a wide variety of symptoms. Everyone has the yeast bug in their gut in harmless quantities (*candida albicans*), but in many people it gets triggered into rapid growth, producing toxins which then affect us, often without our realizing.

A few of the symptoms are of the emotional, mental and physical variety. These are also often 'allergic' type symptoms.

The more obvious yeast conditions are thrush in the vagina or in the mouth, cystitis, abdominal bloating and flatulence.

Many PMS symptoms seem to be aggravated by the yeast bug, *candida*. The vague symptoms of confusion, fatigue, lethargy, depression, poor memory, the feeling of 'not really being there' etc. – the list seems endless.

There are several actions that can be taken to prevent this problem continuing.

Avoiding yeast in food

It is surprising how many foods contain yeast. Yeast is used frequently in food preparation processes, in which case it is generally marked on the label of the product. However, yeast is a fungus which grows on food, particularly left-over food, even if well covered. It is also particularly fond of foods with an acid base like citrus fruits and vinegar.

The following list is a guide to foods high in yeast, which you should try to avoid if you want to reduce the PMS symptoms mentioned above.

1. All foods containing sugar or honey, as yeast thrives on sugary or starchy food.

2. All bread, buns, biscuits, cakes etc.

3. Most alcoholic drinks often depend on yeasts to produce the alcohol, especially beer.

4. Citrus fruit juices – only fresh home-squeezed juice is yeast-free.

5. Malted cereals, malted drinks.

6. Pickles, sauerkraut, olives, chilli peppers.

7. Blue cheese (Roquefort).

8. Mushrooms and mushroom sauce.

9. Hamburgers, sausages and cooked meats made with bread or bread-crumbs. Yeast extract (Miso).

10. All fermented foods.

11. Dried fruits.

12. Left-over or stale food.

13. Vitamins. All B-vitamin preparations are likely to be derived from yeast unless otherwise stated; but most manufacturers do make some B-vitamin preparations which are free of yeasts.

Other contributory factors

Apart from dietary changes there are a few other areas to check. The Pill can make yeast problems worse and should be avoided. Advice should be sought from the Family Planning Clinic for an alternative method of contraception. If the symptoms persist you may need to consult your doctor.

Hints for beating thrush

- Wear cotton underwear instead of nylon.

- Douche with live yoghurt for immediate relief.

- Get your sexual partner treated as well, as it is highly likely that you would pass it back and forwards to each other.

There are some very helpful books on the subject of yeast problems on page 274.

SONIA'S CONTINUING THRUSH SAGA

Sonia is a 39-year-old computer operator with two children. She has been suffering from PMS for many years and her symptoms became severe following the birth of her children. She attended the WNAS clinic at The Nuffield Hospital in Huddersfield.

'When my husband read about the work of the WNAS in the paper, he threw his wallet at me and insisted I make an appointment to attend the

clinic. It got to the point where he wanted to send me away for a week each month as he was so fed up with my behaviour. He simply wasn't prepared to put up with it any more.

I wasn't a nice person

Since the birth of my children my PMS had gradually become worse to the point where I didn't consider myself to be a nice person. My children aren't naughty but at my PMS time I didn't want to see them. I couldn't cope with the hassle. The only way my husband could cope was to go out of the house in order to keep away from me.

In addition to this, following my sterilization last February, I developed severe pain at ovulation time and my periods were so painful each month and so heavy that I had to go to bed for at least a day and drug myself up with painkillers which seemed to make the constipation, which had always been a problem, even worse. In my pre-menstrual week I would binge on chocolate and chocolate biscuits. Looking back I don't know how I managed to eat so much as I was eating meals as well.

I felt reassured to learn that there was a solution to PMS but if I am honest, when I left after my first appointment clutching my recommendations I felt very sceptical. I couldn't believe I would be cured from something I had suffered with for so long. I began my new diet programme, started to exercise regularly and took the supplements that were suggested. I had to keep daily diet diaries and symptom charts and was due to go back for my next appointment four weeks later.

By the time my second consultation arrived I was amazed that I was feeling so much better. My symptoms had vastly reduced to the point where I wouldn't have believed it was possible. My constipation had completely gone, the thrush had cleared up, I managed to keep off chocolate completely and my family were looking hopeful.

By the time I reached my third consultation I was feeling like a completely new person. I have lost 5 kg (11 lb) since starting the programme without dieting and now weigh a trim 54 kg (8 st 8 lb) which meant I had to go shopping for new clothes!

It is four months since I started the programme. My husband can't believe the result after all the years of misery. I am not snarling at the kids any more, I am much more relaxed, I have no need to take painkillers as my periods are no longer painful. My skin is a better colour and it is so soft and clear. I have managed to cope with decorators in the house for the last few months which would have previously resulted in me tearing my hair out. No one who knows me well can believe the transformation. I have got back my self esteem and my husband is just delighted with the result. The solution seems so simple now, we can't believe we have gone on suffering for so long. Our house is now a happy house for the first time in many years and we are all immensely grateful.

I used to get thrush regularly – two or three days each month – which meant I was a regular visitor at my GP surgery. I needed a prescription each month to clear up the dreadfully painful and uncomfortable symptoms. This pattern persisted for at least two years and made me dread my period even more. Amazingly, I haven't had thrush at all since I started on the programme, even in the first month. I have even got to the point where I have forgotten I had it.'

SALLY'S THRUSH PROBLEMS

Sally was a 43-year-old headmistress who also had two young children of her own. She had been diagnosed as having thrush in her oesophagus which was causing her great pain in the chest, particularly on waking.

I had so many problems

'I had continuous digestive problems which had become progressively worse. My doctor had sent me for investigations. I had an endoscopy, where a telescope is passed into the stomach, and a gall-bladder scan, which were clear except for the thrush that was found in my gullet. My worst problem was the extreme pain I experienced on waking each day, and the indigestion. I also had an itchy bottom, so I presumed the thrush went right through my gut. Pre-menstrually I felt angry and clumsy and had experienced very sore breasts.

My job had become very stressful. I couldn't get on top of it somehow. To make matters worse I had developed panic attacks which I thought would subside during the school holidays, but they didn't. My libido had also disappeared and sexual intercourse had become painful as my muscles seemed so tight. A friend had recommended I consult a cranial osteopath for my back problem, and as luck would have it he referred me to the WNAS for help with my other problems.

I was desperate

I was quite sceptical about diet being the solution to what seemed to be extreme symptoms, but I was so desperate that I was willing to try anything, so I went along for an initial consultation, which was very probing. I came away with a programme to start on which involved following an exclusion *diet, particularly wheat, foods that contain yeast, caffeine and alcohol. Plus I was asked to exercise and take some nutritional supplements.*

At my second consultation, which was six weeks later, I was able to report that the pain on waking was only minor and had only occurred once in the last month. My itchy tail had cleared up, my period arrived unannounced with no symptoms or bloating and I felt that I was on the right track. I continued to make progress on all fronts, until Christmas. I was feeling so much better that I went for dried fruit, chocolate, orange juice and wine. The symptoms of thrush flared up and it took a couple of weeks to calm down again, but it really brought home to me how sensitive my body was to these foods and drinks.

I am now back to my old self once more

I have taken up jogging again, which I used to love, and I feel wonderful. All my gut symptoms have disappeared, I no longer feel like I have thrush. My PMS has gone and I am coping really well with situations at work and at home. We have been juggling with my diet for the last six months, and I have gradually been able to add things back without seeing a return of symptoms. I feel very confident that I can manage my health myself now with my new knowledge, and be there for all those who depend upon me.'

SECTION 3: HEADACHES

Do you suffer from the following?

Migraine headaches? ☐

Regular pre-menstrual headaches? ☐

" Melanie's Story "

Melanie was a 39-year-old mother of a teenager who worked full time as a civil servant. She had been suffering from pre-menstrual headaches and sugar cravings for almost three years before she approached the WNAS. They had been bringing her life to a standstill.

'I used to describe myself as the green-eyed monster and covinced myself that nobody cared about how I was feeling in the week before my period, even though I knew this was not true. My husband had been very supportive but

MELANIE

SYMPTOMS

	WEEK AFTER PERIOD (Fill in 3 days after period)				WEEK BEFORE PERIOD (Fill in 2-3 days before period)			
	None	Mild	Moderate	Severe	None	Mild	Moderate	Severe
PMS - A								
Nervous Tension		✓					✓	
Mood Swings		✓					✓	
Irritability			✓					✓
Anxiety			✓					✓
PMS - H								
*Weight Gain	✓					✓		
Swelling of Extremities	✓					✓		
Breast Tenderness	✓						✓	
Abdominal Bloating	✓						✓	
PMS - C								
Headache		✓						✓
Craving for Sweets			✓					✓
Increased Appetite			✓					✓
Heart Pounding	✓				✓			
Fatigue	✓						✓	
Dizziness or Fainting	✓				✓			
PMS - D								
Depression	✓					✓		
Forgetfulness	✓						✓	
Crying	✓					✓		
Confusion	✓					✓		
Insomnia	✓				✓			
OTHER SYMPTOMS								
Loss of Sexual Interest	✓					✓		
Disorientation	✓				✓			
Clumsiness	✓					✓		
Tremors/Shakes	✓				✓			
Thoughts of Suicide	✓				✓			
Agoraphobia	✓				✓			
Increased Physical Activity		✓				✓		
Heavy/Aching Legs	✓					✓		
Generalized Aches	✓					✓		
Bad Breath	✓				✓			
Sensitivity to Music/Light	✓				✓			
Excessive Thirst	✓					✓		

Do you have any other PRE-MENSTRUAL SYMPTOMS not listed above?

1. _____

2. _____

3. _____

4. _____

*5. How much weight do you gain before your period? <u>a few pounds</u>

195

FOLLOW UP
PRE-MENSTRUAL SYNDROME QUESTIONNAIRE

Name: Melanie   Age: 35   Height: 5' 6"   Weight: 10st 0lb

MARITAL STATUS: Single _____   Married ✓   Divorced _____   Widowed _____

(Please tick where applicable)

PRESENT CONTRACEPTION: None _____   Pill _____   I.U.D _____   Other _____

Your periods come every __28__ days   Your periods last __5__ days

Your periods are: Light _____   Moderate ✓   Heavy _____

SYMPTOMS	WEEK AFTER PERIOD (Fill in 3 days after period)				WEEK BEFORE PERIOD (Fill in 2-3 days before period)			
	None	Mild	Moderate	Severe	None	Mild	Moderate	Severe
PMS - A								
Nervous Tension	✓				✓			
Mood Swings	✓				✓			
Irritability	✓				✓			
Anxiety	✓				✓			
PMS - H								
*Weight Gain	✓				✓			
Swelling of Extremities	✓				✓			
Breast Tenderness	✓				✓			
Abdominal Bloating	✓				✓			
PMS - C								
Headache	✓				✓			
Craving for Sweets	✓				✓			
Increased Appetite	✓				✓			
Heart Pounding	✓				✓			
Fatigue	✓				✓			
Dizziness or Fainting	✓				✓			
PMS - D								
Depression	✓				✓			
Forgetfulness	✓				✓			
Crying	✓				✓			
Confusion	✓				✓			
Insomnia	✓				✓			
OTHER SYMPTOMS								
Loss of Sexual Interest	✓				✓			
Disorientation	✓				✓			
Clumsiness	✓				✓			
Tremors/Shakes	✓				✓			
Thoughts of Suicide	✓				✓			
Agoraphobia	✓				✓			
Increased Physical Activity	✓				✓			
Heavy/Aching Legs	✓				✓			
Generalized Aches	✓				✓			
Bad Breath	✓				✓			
Sensitivity to Music/Light	✓				✓			
Excessive Thirst	✓				✓			

regardless of this I was convinced he couldn't care less. My headaches and my nausea were so severe that I had to take three days off work each month and just go to bed as I was unable to function. I would get extremely jealous of my husband and son because they would carry on doing the things that they enjoyed, and I couldn't involve myself because of feeling so unwell. I really felt so frustrated that I was missing out.

Sugar cravings

I experienced really awful sugar cravings. In the week before my period I would be eating three or four bars a day. I had to have chocolate in the house. Even though sometimes I wouldn't eat it, it was comforting to know it was available. What was worse, I would put on around an extra two pounds a month at this time because of this. It would boost my sugar levels, and then I'd feel really fatigued in the few days leading up to my period. Once I was on the WNAS programme chocolate and sweet things were banned. I added far more fresh fruit and vegetables to my diet and increased my physical activity, and at last I was out of that awful spiral of highs and lows.

I'd vow next month would be different

My PMS made life so miserable each month. I would get myself worked up a week before my period was due, wondering if the headaches and nausea would be as bad as the previous month. I worried constantly about how it was affecting my family as I would sometimes say such hurtful things to them and then feel extremely bad afterwards. I was unable to plan anything just in case I had to cancel at the last minute. I was extremely embarrassed at having to explain why I was taking two or three days off work each month.

On good days, after my period arrived, I would go to great lengths to make amends to my family, my friends and my colleagues, all of whom I'd been particularly nasty to in my pre-menstrual phase. I would vow to myself that next month would be different, but inevitably it wasn't.

Changing my lifestyle

Some friends told me about the WNAS and I then happened to read an article in Marie Claire magazine about its work. In desperation I contacted them for some help. As I was too far away from their nearest clinic I enrolled on the telephone and postal consultation service, completed the questionnaire and diet diary and made my first appointment. During my first consultation it was suggested that I make quite considerable dietary changes. Chocolate was definitely banned. I cut out all sorts of foods and drinks and included *lots more fresh fruit and vegetables into my diet, plus I increased my physical activity. In addition to this I took some supplements of Optivite, Efamol and Normoglycaemia to help with my chocolate cravings. I kept diet diaries and symptom charts and had a follow-on consultation at monthly intervals. I began my programme at the end of May and by August practically all my symptoms had gone including the bloating which I didn't even know was associated with PMS.*

I feel my general lifestyle has improved significantly. I no longer feel anxious about what next month will bring and feel more able to cope as the severe headaches have subsided. I enjoy more family time with my husband and son and feel better in myself physically and mentally.'

The green-eyed monster has been replaced by a normal wife and mother who is no longer anxious, preoccupied and sick.

Migraine symptoms may be aggravated by cheese, alcohol, oranges, tea, coffee, chocolate, fermented foods, potted foods and pastes, yeast and wholemeal (wholewheat) bread, smoked and preserved food and yeast extract. It is therefore advisable to avoid these foods where possible for at least a period of two to three months to see whether it makes any difference to your symptoms.

Make sure any vitamin supplements you take are yeast-free.

When you feel a headache coming try chewing some ginger, either crystallized or root. We have a tremendous success rate with migraine.

SECTION 4: SUGAR CRAVINGS

Do you suffer with excessive sugar cravings? There are several things you can do if sugar cravings are a problem.

- Sugar cravings could well improve by taking particular supplements, including vitamin B complex, magnesium and the mineral chromium. Chromium deals with sugar balance in the body, and thus plays an important and effective role in controlling sugar cravings.

- Eat a diet rich in foods containing chromium, magnesium and B vitamins as all of these nutrients have been shown to be necessary for normal blood sugar control. (See page 155).

- Whilst you are experiencing the sugar cravings, eat little and often. In other words, have five or six smaller meals per day, rather than three larger ones. This will help your blood sugar to remain constant and prevent you from having the extreme sugar cravings.

- If sugar cravings are your main problem you may need to refer to another book called *Every Woman's Health Guide*. Details about this book can be found on page 275.

SECTION 5: IRON DEFICIENCY

Do you suffer with the following?

Heavy periods ☐	Cracking at the corners of the mouth	☐
Fatigue ☐	A sore tongue	☐

Heavy periods alone can cause iron deficiency. The other symptoms mentioned above may serve to confirm this. IUDs can sometimes cause heavy bleeding, so if you have a coil, it might be advisable to have a check-up and possibly consider an alternative method of contraception.

With any of the above symptoms you would be wise to ask your doctor to check your serum Ferritin, to see whether you may need some iron supplements. This is a more accurate test of iron stores than haemoglobin. In the meantime you should concentrate on eating iron-rich foods (see page 161).

SECTION 6: ZINC DEFICIENCY

Do you suffer with any of the following?

Acne ☐	Eczema	☐
White spots on your nails ☐	Poor hair growth	☐
Split brittle nails ☐	Infertility	☐
Low libido ☐		

Any combination of the above symptoms may indicate that you need to increase your intake of zinc. This can be done by concentrating on foods rich in zinc and initially by taking a zinc supplement (see page 135).

SECTION 7: FATTY ACID DEFICIENCY

Do you have any of the following?

Dry rough pimply skin on the upper arms or thighs	☐	Dandruff	☐
Red greasy skin	☐	Dry flaky skin	☐
		Eczema	☐

These symptoms may indicate that you are short of essential fatty acids. If you feel this may be so, you can refer to the Food List on essential fats on page 163. Evening primrose oil capsules may be helpful, as is cold pressed linseed oil when taken orally.

SECTION 8: BREAST TENDERNESS

Do you suffer with severe breast tenderness or lumpy breasts pre-menstrually? There are a number of preventive measures you can take:

- Eat a low salt diet.

- Cut out tea and coffee.

- Cut out cigarettes, or at least cut down.

- Restrict your dairy produce intake.

- Keep alcohol consumption to a minimum.

- If taking the contraceptive pill it might be worth changing your Pill or using an alternative method of contraception.

- Take daily supplements of Efamol evening primrose oil (see page 205).

TAKE ONE STEP AT A TIME

There are many new ideas for you to absorb. If you don't feel you can make the necessary changes all at once, then make them gradually. The closer you follow the recommendations, the better off you are likely to feel after you have overcome any withdrawal symptoms that may occur at the very beginning.

It's quite normal to feel sceptical about the value of making such drastic changes. It is only when you start to feel better that you are likely to believe that this is a workable solution.

WILL YOU BE ON A RESTRICTED DIET FOR EVER?

There seems to be a definite difference between a 'food allergy' and a 'food sensitivity'. More often than not we find that severe PMS cases are suffering with food sensitivity rather than actual allergy, although there are cases where women are violently allergic to certain types of food.

Realistically, if you are suffering with severe symptoms, you need to give your body a complete rest for a minimum of two to three months. We often find it takes as much as six months to a year before the body is really back to normal, and can once again cope fully with foods that have been eliminated.

If you notice unpleasant side-effects occurring when you begin to re-introduce the grains, one by one, or products containing yeast, discontinue them for another month or two, before attempting to reintroduce them again. Usually, the very fact that there is so much progress occurring is an incentive to continue with the nutritional programme.

Occasionally we have found that some unfortunate souls have what seems to be a permanent allergy to a particular food, which when reintroduced continues to make them feel very unwell. In these cases the women themselves usually decide that it is better to be well and do without the food in question than to suffer the symptoms.

Once your symptoms are under control it is probably better not to re-introduce foods to your diet during your pre-menstrual week. I usually suggest waiting until your period is over and you are feeling at your best.

CHEATING

One for one, the women who go through the programme cheat at some point. Not only do we expect it, we also think it is a positive step. It's only when you have put the system to the test yourself that you really begin to follow it because you believe in it, rather than following it because someone else said it might work.

I have to smile when I think of the stories I'm told about broken diets. I've been through restricted diets myself, so I know what happens. It goes like this. You begin to feel so well on the diet, in fact you've almost forgotten how rotten you felt initially. Amazing how the memory of pain and discomfort evaporates!

You begin to doubt that you really have food sensitivities, perhaps it's just a coincidence that you felt 'unwell' at the time you were eating your favourite restricted food. So you decide to blow the diet. You eat and enjoy one or two days' helpings of the forbidden 'fruit'. Sometimes the symptoms return within an hour or two, sometimes they creep on within a week or so; either way, you have the symptoms back again and you remember what feeling so unwell was like. You now realize that dietary factors and your symptoms are clearly related. So it's back on the diet with a far more self-determined resolution not to cheat!

IN THE LONG TERM

Once you have been following the dietary and supplement recommendations closely for three or four months, and you have noticed substantial improvement, you can then start to relax a bit. As long as you follow the basic recommendations most of the time, the occasional indulgence shouldn't hurt. Make sure it's only occasional to begin with, and preferably not in the pre-menstrual week. As a general rule, supplements should not be necessary in the long term. They should be taken until you feel that your symptoms are well under control. This may take as little as three or four months or as long as nine months to a year.

Occasionally, months after completing your programme, symptoms may recur. Times of great stress and general illness may, in some circumstances place extra nutritional demands on your body and this may bring on some of the old symptoms. Should this happen to you, identify which PMS category they fall into and take the appropriate dietary action. Use your original programme to help you.

Again, as symptoms reduce, gradually return to the maintenance recommendations and reduce the supplements gradually. It is important to do this in stages as abrupt withdrawal can often lead to recurrence of symptoms.

Do remember to take action quickly with any symptoms so that they can be relieved quickly.

STEP 3 – CHOOSING YOUR SUPPLEMENTS

We never advise women to take random supplements without some sort of advice. Our bodies are fairly sensitive mechanisms which have specific needs. Too much of a particular nutrient can cause imbalances and consequently other problems in the long term.

Before considering supplements, have a look at the chart called 'Physical Signs of Vitamin and Mineral Deficiency' on page 204: you might recognize some of the signs of vitamin and mineral deficiency which you have had for years but accepted as being 'normal'.

PHYSICAL SIGNS OF
VITAMIN AND MINERAL DEFICIENCIES

There are several useful supplements that can be tried in conjunction with each other. Assuming your symptoms are fairly severe and you are looking for the most effective treatment I will first suggest the optimum regime to begin on, regardless of cost. I will then go on to discuss cheaper, and finally, still cheaper alternatives. As you decide which supplements to try, make a note of their name and the daily dosage on your personal tailor-made programme.

MULTI-VITAMIN AND MINERAL SUPPLEMENTS

The first and most basic supplement to take is a multi-vitamin and mineral supplement which contains goodly amounts of the essential nutrients mentioned.

The most tried and tested multi-vitamin and mineral supplement for PMS is an American supplement, formulated by Dr Guy Abraham, Optivite for Women. It has been through several American clinical trials and has been shown to raise progesterone levels. It is available in the USA and the UK.

The Women's Nutritional Advisory Service has conducted two trials on Optivite, the results of which are detailed on page 206.

We usually recommend that four tablets be taken per day during the first few months. After this, reduce down to two per day until mid-cycle, increasing to four per day during your pre-menstrual time. Sometimes, in severe cases, six tablets should be taken per day. If your symptoms are moderate, then a lower dosage may be used.

Another multi-vitamin and mineral supplement that performed well in a clinical trial is Femvite. This new supplement is based on WNAS research and is considerably cheaper than Optivite. It is currently available from Nutritional Health (mail order).

There are certain situations when other supplements need to be taken alongside your multi-vitamin and mineral tablets, some of these are listed on the chart on page 205. We particularly chose Efamol evening primrose oil as it is the only evening primrose oil to have been through repeated trials and we know that each new batch is the same as the last.

If you suffer with severe pre-menstrual breast tenderness you should take a six-month course of Efamol which you can buy over the counter or Efamast, which is available on prescription. Either way you will need to take six capsules for the first two weeks of your cycle, increasing to eight capsules from mid-cycle until the onset of your period. It is advisable to split the dose between breakfast and lunch each day, and to begin by taking one or two capsules for the first few days and gradually building up your dose over a few days.

PHYSICAL SIGNS OF
VITAMIN AND MINERAL DEFICIENCY

Sign or Symptom	Can be Caused by Deficiencies of:
Cracking at the corners of the mouth	Iron, vitamins B12, B6, Folic acid
Recurrent mouth ulcers	Iron, vitamins B12, B6, Folic acid
Dry, cracked lips	Vitamin B2
Smooth (sore) tongue	Iron, vitamins B2, B12, Folic acid
Enlargement/prominence of taste buds at tip of the tongue (red, sore)	Vitamins B2, or B6
Red, greasy skin on face, especially sides of nose	Vitamins B2, B6, zinc or essential fatty acids
Rough, sometimes red, pimply skin on upper arms and thighs	Vitamin B complex, vitamin E or essential fatty acids
Skin conditions such as eczema, dry, rough, cracked, peeling skin	Zinc, essential fatty acids
Poor hair growth	Iron or zinc
Dandruff	Vitamin C, vitamin B6, zinc, essential fatty acids
Acne	Zinc
Bloodshot, gritty, sensitive eyes	Vitamins A or B2
Night blindness	Vitamin A or zinc
Dry eyes	Vitamin A, essential fatty acids
Brittle or split nails	Iron, zinc or essential fatty acids
White spots on nails	Zinc
Pale appearance due to anaemia	Iron, vitamin B12, Folic acid, essential to consult your doctor

Problem	Type of Supplement	Daily Dosage	Available from
*PMS, A, H, C, D	Optivite or Femvite	2–6 tabs daily	Healthfood shops and Nutritional Health (mail order)
*Breast problems	Efamol/Efamast evening primrose oil	4–8 500 mg capsules daily	Chemists, healthfood shops, Nutritional Health (mail order) and prescription
	Natural Vitamin E	400 IUs daily	
Extreme nervous tension, drug withdrawals	Strong Vitamin B complex	1–2 tabs daily	Healthfood shops
*Sugar cravings	Normoglycaemia/ Sugar Factor	1–2 tabs daily	Nutritional Health (mail order)
*Eczema	Efamol/Epogam evening primrose oil	4–8 500 mg tabs daily	Boots, chemists, healthfood shops, (mail order) and prescription
Dry, rough skin/ dandruff	Cold pressed linseed oil	2 tbsp with fruit juice at night	Healthfood shops
*Period pains/ palpitations, insomnia	Magnesium chelate or magnesium hydroxide mixture	2 500 mg tabs daily or 15 ml taken as 5 ml 3 times daily	Healthfood shops and chemists, Nutritional Health (mail order)

*Available by mail order through Nutritional Health, PO Box 926, Lewes, East Sussex BN7 2QL.

IMPORTANT POINTS

- Never take supplements without the consent of your GP if you have a current medical problem.

- Always begin taking your supplements gradually. For example, if you are due to take two or four per day of a particular supplement, begin taking them one tablet per day and gradually build up to the optimum dosage over the period of a week or two. Take them after meals unless otherwise specified.

How to cut down on your supplements

- Cut down on the dosage very gradually over a period of months rather than weeks, but keep taking the supplements each day of your cycle.

- Once you have reduced the dosage gradually, if you feel that your symptoms are well under control you can leave the supplements off altogether the week after your period.

- After another couple of months you can remain supplement-free for two weeks after your period.

- You might prefer to keep taking supplements pre-menstrually, or to cut them out completely and only take them at times of great stress. Some women prefer to take small doses daily on a permanent basis. There is no harm in doing so. As you will probably recognize from Chapter 11, which deals with our diet today, the nutrients in our food are often lost to us, therefore taking supplements in the long term as a general health aid may be a sensible move.

RESULTS OF CLINICAL TRIALS PERFORMED BY THE PRE-MENSTRUAL TENSION ADVISORY SERVICE

Name and type of product	Available from	Dosage given	Improved a lot	Improved slightly	No worse but no better
Optivite	Nature's Best	4 per day increasing to 8 per day pre-menstrually	71.5%	16.5%	12%
Optivite	Nature's Best	2 per day increasing to 4 pre-menstrually	65%	31%	6%
Evening primrose oil (Efamol)	Healthfood shops	8 x 500 mg capsules per day	64%	19%	17%
Femvite	Nutritional Health (mail order)	2 per day	84%	7%	7%
PMT	Australia New Zealand Singapore	2 per day	60%	30%	10%

Out of all the supplements available, only Optivite and Efamol have shown consistently significant results in clinical trials. For details of supplements available in Australia and New Zealand see Appendix 3.

WHAT ABOUT YOUR DRUGS?

If you are currently taking prescribed drugs from your doctor, I don't advise you to stop taking them or reduce them without his or her consent. Having said that, we do find that most women, once established on their nutritional programme, no longer feel the need for their tranquillizers, anti-depressants, sleeping pills or hormone preparations.

Vitamins and minerals can be taken quite happily alongside most drugs. There are a few exceptions however. Any antibiotic in the tetracycline family should not be taken with minerals. Evening primrose oil should not be taken by anyone who has a history of epilepsy. When you feel the time has come to reduce your drugs, do go to see your doctor before taking any action, especially if you have been taking the drugs for a long period of time. Coming off drugs suddenly may bring on nasty withdrawal symptoms.

17

NUTRITIOUS
RECIPES

Although this is not designed to be a recipe book, I felt it would be useful for you to have some guidelines to work with. It's better if you are not short of ideas to begin with: the more you like your new diet, the higher the chances of your sticking to it. In the Recommended Reading List on page 274, I have suggested many inexpensive recipe books which will give you further ideas. It might be an idea to visit a good bookshop and have a browse through the books, so that you can select those you find most suitable.

The recipes I have given cover breakfast, soups, lunch, dinner and sweets. All the recipes are suitable for those of you who are moderate sufferers. For those of you who suffer severely and therefore select a restricted diet, follow the recipes with a code beside them.

There are three codes:

W = Wheat-free.

WOBR = Wheat Oats Barley Rye

Y = Low yeast content.

No code = Suitable for all sufferers who are not on restricted diets.

Note: Imperial and American measures are given in brackets, where appropriate.

Use salt substitute, not salt.

Miso when not in brackets is soya.

BREAKFASTS

WHOLEWHEAT PANCAKES (CREPES)

110 g (4 oz/½ cup) wholemeal
(wholewheat or buckwheat) flour
1 small egg

300 ml (10 fl oz/1¼ cups) skimmed
(skim) milk
oil for cooking

Make a thin batter with the flour, egg and skimmed milk, whisking well. Use kitchen paper to wipe a small non-stick frying pan with oil and heat until it is smoking. Pour a generous 2 tablespoons of the batter into the pan and swirl it around to cover bottom as thinly as possible. Cook the batter for 60 seconds, then flip it over with a spatula and cook the other side for a few seconds only. If you are going to eat straight away, tip on to a heated plate – otherwise, stacked pancakes with cling film (plastic wrap) in between can be stored in the refrigerator. They can be easily reheated individually on a plate covered with foil over a pan of water, or in the microwave oven. SERVES 4

MUESLI

½ mug (½ cup) dried apricots
½ mug (½ cup) jumbo oats
½ mug (½ cup) barley flakes
¼ mug (¼ cup) large sultanas
(golden raisins)

½ pint (1 cup) fresh orange juice
2 apples, grated
milk to mix
¼ mug (¼ cup) chopped mixed nuts
clear honey, to taste

Put apricots, oats, barley flakes, sultanas and orange juice in a mixing bowl. Cover and leave to soak overnight. Next morning, stir in the apple and sufficient milk to give a soft consistency. Spoon the muesli into dishes and top with chopped nuts and honey. SERVES 3–4

ALTERNATIVE MUESLI WOBR

1 mug (1 cup) Cornflakes
1 mug (1 cup) Puffed Wheat
½ mug (½ cup) sunflower seeds
½ mug (½ cup) chopped almonds

½ mug (½ cup) chopped pecan nuts
½ mug (½ cup) organic raisins
½ mug (½ cup) chopped apricots
⅓ mug (⅓ cup) pine nuts

Chop the apricots, almonds and pecan nuts. Mix together with the dry ingredients and raisins. I usually recommend making a larger quantity and storing in a sealed container. NB: Serve with chopped fresh fruit, a little bio yoghurt and semi-skimmed milk. If constipated add 2 tablespoons of linseeds to each serving. SERVES 6–8

HOT FRUITY BREAKFAST WOBR

25 g (1 oz/2 tbsp) lightly crushed millet, toasted

150 ml (¼ pint/½ cup) milk stewed fruit according to taste

Mix the millet and milk in a pan. Bring gently to the boil and simmer for 5 minutes, stirring occasionally. Put in a serving bowl, stir in 15–30 ml (1–2 tbsp) stewed fruit, and serve with extra milk substitute or a spoonful of sugar-free jam. SERVES 1

DRIED FRUIT CONSERVE WOBR

200 g (7 oz/1 cup) dried apricots
apple juice
**Use one of the following
  flavourings:**
5 ml (1 tsp) orange flower water

or
5 ml (1 tsp) grated orange peel
or
50 g (2 oz/½ cup) flaked almonds

Soak apricots overnight in water. Put the apricots into a saucepan and just cover them with apple juice, using the minimum amount to ensure a thick pureé. Simmer them, uncovered, for about 30 minutes or until they are thoroughly cooked and soft. Cool and then thoroughly blend or sieve them until they have a smooth, thick consistency. Add one of the flavourings.

Pureé will keep in refrigerator for about 10 days. SERVES 2

SOUPS

LENTIL AND VEGETABLE SOUP WOBR

15 g (½ oz) soft vegetable margarine
1 onion, chopped
1 garlic clove, crushed
2 large carrots, finely diced
2 sticks celery, sliced
2 tomatoes, skinned and chopped
50 g (2 oz/1 cup) mushrooms,
  chopped

100 g (4 oz) cabbage, shredded
100 g (4 oz/½ cup) continental
  lentils, pre-soaked
1 litre (1¾ pints) vegetable stock
bouquet garni (sprig parsley, thyme
  and bay leaf tied)
parsley
pepper

Melt margarine in a large saucepan and sauté the onion for five minutes without browning. Add garlic and rest of vegetables and cook gently for five minutes over the heat, then add the stock and bouquet garni, stir in extra parsley and season to taste with pepper. SERVES 4

BROCCOLI SOUP WOBR&Y

225 g (8 oz–1 lb) broccoli, chopped
1.7 litres (3 pints) vegetable stock
1.25 ml (¼ tsp) salt

30 ml (2 tbsp) semi-skimmed (skim) milk
pinch nutmeg
pinch cayenne pepper

Combine broccoli, stock and salt in large saucepan, bring to the boil. Reduce heat and simmer for 15 minutes. Remove from heat, blend mixture to pureé with milk, nutmeg and cayenne. Return to pan, heat through, do not boil. SERVES 6

NUTTY PARSNIP SOUP WOBR

25 g (1 oz/1 tbsp) vegetable margarine
1 medium onion, chopped
300 g (10½ oz) parsnips, sliced
1 tbsp smooth peanut butter

dash shoyu (soya derivative, from healthfood shops)
1 vegetable stock cube
600 ml (1 pint) water
25 g (1 oz/¼ cup) peanuts, roasted

Melt the margarine in a deep pan. Sauté the onions and parsnips together until beginning to soften. Stir in the peanut butter to coat the vegetables. Add a little shoyu. Bring vegetable stock to the boil and add the water gradually, allowing the peanut butter to thicken slightly. Continue cooking until all ingredients are soft. Blend. Roughly grate the peanuts and scatter on the surface just before serving. (Hazelnuts and hazelnut butter can be used instead.) SERVES 4

FRESH AVOCADO AND TOMATO SOUP WOBR&Y

50 g (2 oz/¼ stick) butter/margarine
1 medium-sized onion, chopped
1 small potato, chopped
450 g (1 lb) tomatoes, quartered
2 garlic cloves

1 bay leaf
30 ml (2 tbsp) tomato pureé (paste)
450 ml (¾ pint) vegetable stock
450 ml (¾ pint) milk
2 avocados (ripe)
pepper to taste

Melt the butter/margarine and sauté the onion until transparent. Add potato, tomatoes, garlic, bay leaf, tomato paste and stock. Cover and simmer for 20 minutes. Take off the heat, stirring in the milk and chopped avocado flesh. Remove bay leaf. Blend in small quantities in liquidizer goblet. Adjust seasoning to taste and reheat to serving temperature. SERVES 4–6

CHICKEN SOUP WOBR&Y

1 chicken boned and cut into 2.5 cm (1 in) cubes
600 ml (1 pint) water
4 garlic cloves, sliced (optional, to taste)
2 sticks of celery, chopped

2 carrots, chopped
1 medium onion
50 g (2 oz) peas
50 g (2 oz) cooked brown rice
25 g (1 oz) parsley, chopped
herbs and seasoning to taste

Simmer chicken in water for 40 minutes. Add garlic, vegetables and rice and simmer for additional 20 minutes. Serve topped with scissor-snipped fresh parsley. Add herbs according to taste. SERVES 4

SALADS

Always use the very best and freshest ingredients.

BEANSHOOT SALAD WOBR&Y

50 g (2 oz/½ cup) almond halves
1 tsp oil
¼ tsp salt

50 g (2 oz) carrots
2 bananas
300 g (8 oz) fresh beanshoots

Put the almonds, oil and salt in small ovenproof dish. Mix well, then roast in the oven at 200°C (400°F/Mark 6) for about 10 minutes until golden. Leave until cold. Grate carrots and slice the bananas, combine with almonds and beanshoots. SERVES 4

WALDORF SALAD WOBR

4 sticks celery
50 g (2 oz/½ cup) walnuts
1 large dessert apple

150 g (6 oz) Cheddar cheese
salt and pepper
French dressing

Chop the celery and walnuts. Dice the apple and cheese. Mix all the

ingredients together in a salad bowl. Add seasoning and dressing to taste.
SERVES 4

BULGAR AND NUT SALAD

200 g (8 oz/1⅓ cups) bulgar
   (cracked wheat)
1 large sized onion, finely chopped
3 tbsp olive oil
100 ml (4 fl oz) tomato pureé
   (paste)
60 ml (4 tbsp) dried mint

5 ml (1 tsp) ground cumin
5 ml (1 tsp) ground coriander
2.5 ml (½ tsp) ground allspice
110 g (4 oz/1 cup) walnuts and/or
   hazelnuts, very coarsely chopped
juice of 1 lemon

Soak the cracked wheat (available from healthfood shops) in plenty of
fresh cold water for 15 minutes, drain it well and squeeze out as much of
the water as you can. Fry the chopped onion in a tablespoon of oil, until
very soft but not yet coloured. Mix all the ingredients in a large serving
bowl and leave for about an hour for the bulgar to absorb the flavours and
become plump and tender. SERVES 4

GRAPEFRUIT AND ORANGE SALAD WOBR&Y

1 whole grapefruit
1 orange
75 g (3 oz/½ cup) sunflower seeds

50 g (2 oz/½ cup) mixed nuts
   chopped
orange juice, freshly squeezed

Remove rind of grapefruit and orange and chop flesh, mix with sunflower
seeds and nuts and a little orange juice. SERVES 4

ORANGE AND CUCUMBER SALAD WOBR&Y

2 oranges, divided into segments
½ cucumber, thinly sliced

1 small onion, thinly sliced into rings
½ small lettuce

Mix all ingredients together. SERVES 4

GREEN BEAN AND SWEETCORN SALAD WOBR&Y

200 g (8 oz) young French beans,
   topped and tailed
150 g (6 oz) can sweetcorn

2 spring onions (scallions), thinly
   sliced
2 tbsp French dressing (not for low
   yeast diet)

Cook the beans in slightly salted boiling water until tender. Drain, refresh in cold running water, leave to cool. Mix together the beans, sweetcorn and onions, Stir together with French dressing. SERVES 4

SALAD DRESSINGS

PEANUT AND CHILLI WOBR

25 ml (1 fl oz/2 tbsp) peanut oil
1 medium onion, thinly sliced
2.5 ml (½ tsp) chilli powder
5 ml (1 tsp) sugar/honey
5 ml (1 tsp) shoyu/tamari (soy sauce, from healthfood shops)
15 ml (1 tbsp) tomato pureé (paste) (optional)

30–45 ml (2–3 tbsp) peanut butter (smooth)
3 cloves garlic, crushed or finely chopped
200 ml (7 fl oz/1 cup) water
200 ml (7 fl oz/1 cup) milk
dash of pepper

Heat oil gently and stir in onion, chilli, sugar/honey and shoyu, cook until onion is soft. Stir in tomato pureé, peanut butter and garlic. Add water and milk and bring back to the boil, stirring regularly until mixture is smooth and not too thick. Season with pepper to taste.

It is important that the consistency is not too thick as it will become thick and lumpy if overcooked. MAKES 2½ CUPS

AVOCADO AND YOGHURT DRESSING WOBR&Y

1 ripe avocado
½ lemon
400 ml (14 fl oz) yoghurt

3 cloves garlic (crushed)
pinch of salt and pepper

Halve the avocado and scoop out the flesh, blend or mash immediately with lemon juice. Fold yoghurt and garlic into avocado mixture until smooth. Season to taste, or season with chilli or cayenne pepper. MAKES 2½ CUPS

YOGHURT HERB DRESSING WOBR

125 ml (5 fl oz/½ cup) natural yoghurt
1 clove garlic, crushed
15 ml (1 tbsp) cider vinegar

5 ml (1 tsp) clear honey
15 g (½ oz) parsley
15 g (½ oz) mixed mint and herbs
pinch of salt and pepper

Place all ingredients except herbs in a bowl, adding salt and pepper to taste and mix thoroughly with a fork. Add herbs finely chopped and mix well or blend for 1–2 minutes. Chill until required. MAKES 1 CUP

CREAMY TOMATO DRESSING WOBR&Y

30 ml (2 tbsp) home-made
   mayonnaise
1 tomato, chopped

10 ml (2 tsp) lemon juice
2.5 ml (½ tsp) dried or 1 tsp fresh
   basil

Blend all the ingredients together on low speed. MAKES ABOUT ⅓ CUP

OIL AND FRUIT DRESSING WOBR

30 ml (2 tbsp) olive oil
15 ml (1 tbsp) sesame oil
5 ml (1 tsp) mayonnaise
5 ml (1 tsp) mustard

juice from a lemon or 15 ml (1 tbsp)
   wine vinegar
5 ml (1 tsp) concentrated apple juice
   (optional)
black pepper to taste

Blend all the ingredients together until smooth. This dressing keeps well in the fridge in a sealed container. MAKES 1 CUP

LUNCHES AND DINNERS

GRILLED (BROILED) SARDINES WOBR&Y

Wash and dry sardines, dust with peppered flour (non-wheat flour for restricted diets) and grill (broil) for 5–10 minutes depending on size, turning once.
or
Place sardines on the grill (broiler), sprinkle with pepper and olive oil and grill for 5–10 minutes depending on size, turning once.

STUFFED PEPPERS WOBR

1 medium onion
2 sticks celery
100 g (4 oz) mushrooms
1 large tomato
1 medium-sized carrot
25 g (1 oz/½ stick) margarine
100 ml (5 fl oz/½ cup) water
5 ml (1 tsp) tomato pureé (paste)

2.5 ml (½ tsp) yeast extract (Miso)
4 medium-size green or red (bell)
    peppers
30 ml (2 tbsp) buckwheat or other
    grain-free flour
seasoning to taste
100 g (4 oz) Cheddar cheese, grated

Chop the onion, celery, mushrooms and tomatoes and dice the carrot, melt margarine and fry onion, carrot, celery and mushrooms together for 5 minutes. Stir in the tomato, water, tomato pureé and yeast extract. Cover and simmer for 10–15 minutes, until just tender. Meanwhile, halve peppers lengthways and remove the seeds, then steam for 10 minutes. Arrange in an ovenproof serving dish. Drain vegetables, reserving the cooking liquid. Fill the peppers with the vegetables. Sprinkle the flour into the vegetable liquid and bring to the boil. Adjust seasoning to taste. Pour over the peppers, sprinkle with the cheese and bake in the oven at 200° (400°/Mark 6) for 15 minutes. Serve at once. SERVES 4

SPANISH OMELETTE WOBR&Y

1 small onion, chopped
25 ml (1 fl oz/¼ cup) water
1 stick celery, chopped
1 green (bell) pepper

2 eggs
5 ml (1 tsp) butter
2 tomatoes, chopped
parsley (scissor-snipped)

Place the onions and water in a sealed pan over a medium heat. When water begins to boil reduce the heat to low. Add celery and green pepper and continue cooking until soft. Do not overcook. Beat eggs, melt butter in a medium frying pan over a low heat. Pour in beaten eggs and allow to cook gently. Strain vegetables, tip on to partly cooked omelette and add tomatoes. When cooked serve sprinkled with parsley. SERVES 1

STIR-FRY VEGETABLES WOBR†*

There are many different combinations of vegetable in season that can be used for stir-frying. You can use six or seven different vegetables or only two or three.

To obtain the best results, stir-fry vegetables should be cooked with the minimum oil at a high heat as rapid cooking seals in the flavour.

Here are some nice last-minute additions to your stir-fry. Experiment to find your favourite seasoning and flavouring. Less well-known ingredients are available from healthfood shops.

*Seasoning

Salt, pepper, chilli, grated ginger, five spice (use very moderately), sesame seeds (ground), fenugreek (ground), turmeric, coriander, paprika, nori seaweed (toasted and crumbled).

*Flavouring

Shoyu/tamari, Miso (all Japanese/Chinese condiments made from soya beans), sesame oil, tahini (sesame seed butter), sunflower oil, safflower oil, sherry, vermouth, lemon juice.

450 g (1 lb) fresh broccoli	2.5 ml (½ tsp) sesame oil
225 g (8 oz) cauliflower	225 g (8 oz) fresh bean sprouts
15 ml (1 tbsp) oil	225 g (8 oz) Chinese leaves or white
2.5 cm (1 in) fresh ginger, sliced and	cabbage, shredded
finely shredded	2.5 ml (½ tsp) salt
2 large carrots, peeled and sliced	

Separate the broccoli heads into small florets and peel and slice the stems. Separate the cauliflower florets and slice stems. Heat oil in a large wok or frying pan. When it is moderately hot add ginger shreds. Stir-fry for a few seconds. Add the carrots, cauliflower and broccoli and stir-fry for 2–3 minutes then add sesame seed oil, bean sprouts and Chinese leaves or white cabbage. Stir-fry for further 2–3 minutes. Season to taste. Serve at once. SERVES 4–6

*† and Y if yeast-free flavouring selected

Bear in mind that ordinary soya sauce is not wheat free. Use tamari wheat-free soya sauce instead, which is available from healthfood shops.

Ginger can be substituted for garlic and soy sauce can be added in final stage of frying before serving.

MACKEREL WITH HERBS (IN FOIL) WOBR&Y

4 medium-sized fresh mackerel,	4 small bunches of 4 different fresh
gutted	mixed herbs, e.g. tarragon, chives,
juice of one lemon	parsley and sage
freshly ground black pepper	little olive oil

Pre-heat oven to 240°C (475°F/Mark 9). Wash mackerel and sprinkle insides with lemon juice. Add generous sprinkling of pepper. Put bunch of mixed herbs inside each fish and brush skin with oil to avoid sticking, wrap each fish individually in foil, quite tightly, bake for 10–12 minutes and serve. SERVES 4

STUFFED MACKEREL IN FOIL WBR

2 large oranges
4 tbsp porridge (rolled oats)
1 medium-sized onion, finely chopped
1 tbsp parsley, finely chopped
1 tbsp raisins

1 apple, grated
pinch of salt
1 tsp dried rosemary or 4 sprigs fresh
   rosemary
4 medium-sized fresh mackerel, gutted

Grate zest of orange, chop flesh into small pieces, discarding pips and any tough pith. Mix the orange zest and flesh with oats, onion, parsley, raisins and grated apple and pinch of salt. Divide mixture into 4 and stuff mackerel loosely. Place rosemary in each fish. Bake in foil as above for about 40 minutes. SERVES 4

VEGETARIAN GOULASH WOBR

45 ml (3 tbsp) oil
1 medium onion, sliced
2 medium carrots, diced
2 medium courgettes (zucchini),
   sliced
½ small white cabbage, finely
   shredded
15 ml (1 tbsp) paprika

2.5 ml (½ tsp) caraway seeds
2.5 ml (½ tsp) mixed herbs
pinch of nutmeg
600 ml (1 pint) tomato juice
300 ml (½ pint) water
1 vegetable stock cube
142 ml (¼ pint) soured cream or
   natural yoghurt

Heat oil in large saucepan and sauté the onion and carrot until the onion is transparent. Add courgettes and cabbage and cook over medium heat for 10 minutes, stirring frequently. Stir in paprika, caraway seeds, herbs and nutmeg, then add tomato juice, water and stock cube. Cover and simmer for about 20 minutes until the vegetables are just tender. Adjust seasoning with a small pinch salt and pepper. Serve each portion with a drop of soured cream or yogurt. Serve at once. SERVES 4–6

STEAMED FISH (WITH GARLIC, SPRING ONIONS [SCALLIONS] AND GINGER) WOBR

350 g (12 oz) firm white fish fillets
(cod, sole etc)
2.5 ml (½ tsp) salt
15 ml (1 tbsp) fresh ginger, finely
chopped
30 ml (2 tbsp) spring onions
(scallions), finely chopped

15 ml (1 tbsp) tamari wheat-free
soya sauce
15 ml (1 tbsp) oil, preferably
groundnut
5 ml (1 tsp) sesame oil
2 garlic cloves, peeled and thinly
sliced

Rub cleaned and dried fish with salt both sides and leave for 30 minutes. Steam fish over simmering water until just cooked, covering steamer tightly. Sprinkle on the ginger, spring onions and tamari wheat-free soya sauce. Heat the two oils together in small saucepan, when hot add garlic slices and brown. Pour the garlic oil mixture over the top of the fish. Serve at once. SERVES 4

SNOW PEAS WITH TIGER PRAWNS WOBR

450 g (1 lb) snow peas (mange
tout))
450 g (1 lb) uncooked tiger prawns
375 g (13 oz) uncooked broad
oriental rice noodles
5 ml (1 tsp) finely chopped root ginger

45 ml (3 tbsp) sesame oil
30 ml (2 tbsp) oyster sauce
5 ml (1 tsp) sugar
15 ml (1 tbsp) sherry or white wine
fresh coriander to decorate

Top and tail the snow peas and wash them. Clean and wash the prawns and pat them dry with kitchen paper. Place the noodles in boiling water and simmer gently for 3 minutes, until slightly undercooked. Place the ginger and the oil in a wok and heat. Fry the snow peas briefly in the hot oil stirring constantly. Remove and place on a warmed dish. Place the tiger prawns in the wok and cook until they become pink. Drain the noodles and rinse with cold water to remove the starch. Return snow peas to the wok with the prawns, add the oyster sauce and the sugar, and simmer for another minute or two. Gently pour one tablespoon of sherry or white wine around the circumference of the wok, and then remove peas and prawns from the wok with a slatted spoon and transfer to a dish. Place noodles in the wok and quickly stir-fry them in the remaining oil turning constantly. Turn the noodles out onto a flat platter and place the snow peas and prawns on the top. Decorate with fresh coriander and serve immediately. SERVES 4

Variation If you like spicy food, before stir-frying the noodles mix 5 ml (1 tsp) chilli sauce with the hot oil and then place the noodles in the wok.

FRAGRANT LAMB WOBR

2–3 lb (900 g–1.3 kg) fillet joint of
   leg of lamb or 6 fillets of lamb
45 ml (3 tbsp) sesame oil
1 clove of garlic, chopped
1.25 cm (½ in) lump of root ginger,
   chopped
whole spring onion
45 ml (3 tbsp) tamari wheat-free
   soya sauce

30 ml (2 tbsp) brandy
45 ml (3 tbsp) white wine
black pepper to taste or a sprinkling
   of black peppercorns
5 ml (1 flat tsp) cornflour
8 large lettuce leaves to decorate the
   serving plate
sprig of coriander

Seal the lamb by cooking in a little hot sesame oil for two minutes each side. Remove the lamb from the hot oil and place in a pressure cooker. Add the chopped garlic, chopped ginger, the whole spring onion, the remaining sesame oil, soya sauce, brandy, white wine, and black pepper or peppercorns. Put the lid on the pressure cooker and bring to the boil. Lower the heat, and cook at pressure for 35 minutes. Decorate a large serving dish with lettuce leaves ready to receive the lamb. Remove the pressure cooker from the heat and place under cold running water to cool. Place the lamb on a chopping board and slice into portions. Arrange the chops or the sliced lamb joint on the serving dish and place in the oven to keep warm whilst you prepare the sauce. Drain the juice and thicken with the cornflour, stirring constantly. Remove the serving dish from the oven, pour the sauce over the lamb and decorate with the coriander. Serve immediately. SERVES 6

LAMB PAPRIKA WOBR

2 onions, sliced
50 g (2 oz) mushrooms, sliced
2 carrots, sliced
4 lamb chops (lean)

30 ml (2 tbsp) paprika
450 ml (¾ pint) water
15 ml (1 tbsp) cornflour (cornstarch)
   (or alternative grain-free flour)

Mix vegetables together and place in casserole. Arrange chops on top. Stir paprika into water and pour over chops, cover and cook until chops are tender. Remove vegetables and chops and arrange on warm serving dish. Mix cornflour with a little cold water and use to thicken liquid from chops. Cook for 2–3 minutes, pour over chops. SERVES 2–4

LIVER WITH ORANGE WOBR

225 g (8 oz) lamb's liver
30 ml (2 tbsp) wholewheat flour (or
    alternative grain-free flour)
2.5 ml (½ tsp) dried thyme or basil
25 ml (1½ tbsp) sunflower oil

1 orange, peeled and sliced
grated orange peel
15 ml (1 tbsp) tamari wheat-free
    soya sauce
30 ml (2 tbsp) orange juice

Wash liver, slice thinly, pat dry with kitchen paper. Cut out and discard stringy pieces, coat in flour seasoned with herbs. Heat oil in a frying pan and fry liver pieces gently for 5 minutes, turning to cook evenly. Add orange slices and peel, soya sauce and orange juice. Heat through gently and serve. SERVES 2

NUT ROAST WOBR

1 medium onion
25 g (1 oz/¼ stick) butter/margarine
225 g (8 oz/2 cups) mixed nuts
100 g (4 oz/2 cups) cooked brown
    rice

200 ml (½ pint) vegetable stock
10 ml (2 tsp) yeast extract (Miso)
5 ml (1 tsp) mixed herbs
salt and pepper to taste

Chop onions and sauté in butter until transparent. Grind nuts in a blender or food processor until quite fine. Heat stock and yeast extract to boiling point, then combine all the ingredients including the cooked brown rice together and mix well until the mixture is a fairly slack consistency. Turn into greased shallow baking dish, level the surface, and bake in oven at 180°C (350°F/Mark 4) for 30 minutes until golden brown. SERVES 4–6

COLOURFUL LENTILS WOBR

60 ml (4 tbsp) oil
3 cloves garlic, crushed
4 carrots, chopped
1 green (bell) pepper, chopped
1 red (bell) pepper, chopped
5 ml (1 tsp) basil
3 sticks celery, chopped

15 ml (1 tbsp) brown rice miso
900 ml (1½ pints) hot water
675 g (1½ lb) tomatoes, skinned,
    seeded and chopped
280 g (10 oz) lentils, not presoaked
30 ml (2 tbsp) chopped parsley
seasoning to taste

Heat oil in a pan and add the garlic, carrots, green and red peppers, basil and celery. Cook until the ingredients are soft. Mix the brown rice miso with hot water and add this to mixture, together with the tomatoes. Stir in the lentils. Season to taste. Simmer for 1 hour. Serve, garnished with the chopped parsley. SERVES 4 OR 6 AS A STARTER

STUFFING FOR ROAST CHICKEN WOBR

1 stick celery, finely chopped
2 cloves garlic, crushed
30 ml (2 tbsp) sunflower oil
60 g (2 oz/¼ cup) uncooked long
   grain brown rice
150 ml (¼ pint) hot water

120 g (4 oz/2 cups) mushrooms,
   sliced
30 g (1 oz/⅙ cup) sultanas
60 g (2 oz/⅓ cup) dried apricots,
   soaked and chopped
30 ml (2 tbsp) tarragon

Fry the celery and garlic in the oil for 2–3 minutes. Add the rice and sauté for a few minutes. Pour in the hot water, stir, then simmer for 5–6 minutes until most of the water has been absorbed, but the rice is still hard. Remove from the heat and mix in the remaining ingredients. Allow to cool for a little, then use to stuff the chicken.

SWEETS

FRUIT JELLY WOBR

22 g (¾ oz) gelatine
600 ml (1 pint) unsweetened fruit
   juice
   e.g. apple, pineapple

Sprinkle the gelatine on 1 tbsp heated fruit juice and stir well until dissolved. Add the rest of the juice. Put into a wetted mould and chill until set. SERVES 4

DRIED FRUIT COMPOTE AND YOGHURT WOBR

15 g (½ oz/1 tbsp) sugar
600 ml (1 pint) water
5–10 cm (2–3 in) stick of cinnamon

450 g (1 lb) mixed dried fruit e.g.
   apple rings, peaches, apricots,
   prunes, pears and sultanas

Dissolve the sugar in the water over a gentle heat, add the cinnamon. Place the dried fruit in a bowl and pour the syrup over. Cover and leave to soak overnight. If the soaked fruit is not tender, replace in the pan and simmer for a few minutes. Serve cold with yoghurt. SERVES 4–6

RHUBARB FOOL WOBR

25 g (1 oz/¼ stick) margarine
225 g (8 oz) rhubarb

12–25 g (½–1 oz) brown sugar
200 ml (7 fl oz) natural yoghurt

Melt margarine in a pan. Add rhubarb and sugar and cook until tender. Pureé rhubarb and yoghurt together in a blender. Chill before serving. SERVES 4

STUFFED BAKED APPLES WOBR

4 good-sized cooking apples
1 tbsp honey/sugar-free jam

Stuffing suggestions:
Dates, cinnamon, raisins and honey

Core apples and slit skins in a ring round the middle. Stuff with chosen filling and honey. Bake until fruit is tender. Serve hot or cold. SERVES 4

CARROT CAKE WOBR

4 eggs
225 g (8 oz/1 cup) caster (superfine)
   sugar
grated rind of 1 lemon
225 g (8 oz/2 cups) ground almonds

225 g (8 oz) carrots, finely grated
75 g (3 oz) raisins
75 g (3 oz) sultanas
25 ml (1½ tbsp) rice flour
5 ml (1 tsp) wheat-free baking
   powder

Pre-heat the oven to 180°C (350°F/Mark 4). Separate the eggs. Place yolks, sugar and lemon rind in a bowl or in a blender or food processor and beat together well. Add the almonds and carrots to this mixture. Stir well. Sift the flour and baking powder together then fold into mixture. In another bowl beat the egg whites until they are stiff, then fold them into the mixture. Add the dried fruit and stir gently. Grease two oblong loaf tins 19 cm (7½ in) long. Spread the mixture out in the tray and bake for 45 minutes. Leave to cool in the tins, then cut into slices. MAKES 16 SLICES

Optional topping: Mix the juice of a lemon with 50–75 g (2–3 oz) icing sugar until it forms a smooth but runny paste. Drizzle the icing on top of the cool carrot cake and leave to set.

BANANA CREAM WOBR

4 medium bananas
15 ml (1 tbsp) lemon juice

400 ml (15 fl oz/2 cups) yoghurt
5 ml (1 tsp) honey

Place all ingredients in the blender and blend until creamy. Chill well before serving. SERVES 4

FRUITY CAKES WOBR

100 g (4 oz/1 stick) butter/margarine
100 g (4 oz) unrefined sugar
(reduced to caster (superfine)
sugar consistency in a blender or
food processor)
2 eggs, beaten

200 g (5½ oz) Trufree No 7 self-
raising (self-rising) flour, or a
combination of corn and
rice flour
100–150 g (4–6 oz/¾–1 cup) mixed
raisins, currants and sultanas
(golden raisins)

Cream butter or margarine and sugar till light and fluffy. Add eggs gradually then fold in flour. Stir in mixed dried fruit. Put mixture into individual cake cases and bake at 190°C (375°F/Mark 5) for 15–18 minutes till risen and golden.

Alternatively place all the mixture in a 500 g (1 lb) loaf tin and cook at 180°C (350°F/Mark 4) for 20–25 minutes for a sweet fruit loaf. MAKES 10 CAKES

GINGER BANANAS WOBR

4 ripe bananas
small amount preserved ginger

25 g (1 oz) flaked almonds

Slice the bananas into individual dishes (one per person). Rinse the syrup from the preserved ginger and chop fairly finely. Sprinkle ginger over the bananas and top with a few almonds. SERVES 4

Variation Mix in a few drops of lemon juice and sprinkle with sunflower seeds.

EGG CUSTARD WOBR

175 ml (6 fl oz/¾ cup) milk
2 egg yolks
mild honey to taste

a few drops of real vanilla essence
(optional)

Heat the milk to boiling point and add slowly to the well-beaten egg yolks. Return to the pan, preferably a double boiler, and stir over a gentle heat until the mixture thickens slightly. Sweeten to taste with honey and add a

few drops of vanilla essence if liked. The custard will thicken as it cools.
SERVES 2

CAKES, BISCUITS AND BREAD

BUCKWHEAT AND RICE BREAD WOBR

This makes brown bread which is crisp on the outside and soft on the inside.

300 g (12 oz) buckwheat flour	2.5–5 ml (½–1 tbsp) salt
150 g (6 oz) brown rice flour	425 ml (¾ pint) hand-hot
1½ packets easy yeast	water
5 ml (1 tsp) sugar	2 500 g (1 lb) loaf tins
15 ml (1 tbsp) oil	

Mix together flours and easy yeast. Add sugar, oil and salt and mix to a thick batter with the hand-hot water. Grease and flour the two loaf tins. Divide mixture between the two loaf tins, cover and leave to rise in a warm place for 20–30 minutes. Bake at 230°C (450°F/Mark 8) for 35–40 minutes. The bread will slightly contract from the side of the tins when it is cooked. Cool for 5 minutes in the tins and then turn out on to a wire rack. MAKES 14 SLICES (7 EACH LOAF)

POTATO AND RICE BREAD WOBR

This is a white bread which is delicious when freshly baked, and subsequently makes very nice toast. It tastes rather like crumpets.

250 g (10 oz) potato flour	15 ml (1 tbsp) oil
200 g (8 oz) brown rice flour	2.5–5 ml (½–1 tsp) salt
1½ packets easy yeast	425 ml (¾ pint) hand-hot water
5 ml (1 tsp) sugar	2 500 g (1 lb) loaf tins

Mix together flours and easy yeast. Add sugar, oil and salt and mix to a thick batter with the hand-hot water. Grease and flour the two loaf tins. Divide mixture between the two loaf tins, cover and leave to rise in a warm place for 20–30 minutes. Bake at 230°C (450°F/Mark 8) for 35–40 minutes. The bread will contract slightly from the side of the tins when it is cooked. Cool for 5 minutes in the tins and then turn out on to a wire rack. MAKES 16 SLICES (8 EACH LOAF)

POTATO SHORTBREAD WOBR

150 g (6 oz) potato flour
100 g (4 oz) margarine

50 g (2 oz) sugar
75 g (3 oz) ground almonds

Put all ingredients in to a food processor and beat together for 5–6 seconds. Scrape bowl and repeat the process until a ball of dough is formed. Put dough into a greased 7–8 in (17.5–20 cm) round sandwich tin and press down evenly. Mark out portions with a knife, prick all over and bake at 180°C (350°F/Mark 4) for 35–40 minutes. Cut into wedges and cool in tin. MAKES 8 SLICES

APPLE AND CINNAMON CAKE WOBR

4 large cooking apples
100 g (4 oz) brown rice flour
4 large eggs
100 g (4 oz) ground almonds
75 g (3 oz) caster sugar
100 g (4 oz) cooking flora
few drops of almond essence to
    flavour

15 ml (1 tbsp) cinnamon

To decorate:

approximately 16 apple slices
7.5 ml (½ tbsp) cinnamon
15 ml (1 tbsp) caster sugar

Grease a deep 8 in (20 cm) loose-bottomed circular baking tin. Pre-heat oven to moderate temperature, 150°C (300°F/Mark 2). Peel, core and slice the apples and leave to soak in cold water. Place the flour, eggs, ground almonds, caster sugar, cooking flora and almond essence in the bowl of a mixer and beat until light and fluffy. Line the cake tin with approximately 1½ in (3.75 cm) of mixture. Place most of the apples in the tin and sprinkle with sugar and cinnamon. Spread the additional mixture on to the top of the apples and smooth off the top ready for the decoration. Gently push remaining apple slices into the top of the cake in a circle and sprinkle with cinnamon and sugar. Bake in a moderate oven for at least one hour, until cooked through. Cool briefly, then gently ease the cake out of the tin and on to a plate. Serve hot as a pudding or cold as a cake with whipped or pouring cream. MAKES 8 GOOD SIZED SLICES

ALMOND MACAROONS WOBR

2 large egg whites
150 g (6 oz) ground almonds

75 g (3 oz) caster sugar
18 almond halves

Put the unbeaten egg whites into a bowl with the ground almonds, and beat well adding the caster sugar 1 tablespoon at a time. Line biscuit trays with greaseproof paper. With moist hands roll the mixture into balls and flatten in the palm of your hand. Lay the flattened biscuits carefully on to the trays and place an almond half in the middle of each biscuit. Bake in a moderate oven at 180°C (350°F/Mark 4) for 25 minutes or until golden brown. Keep in an airtight tin, or freeze. MAKES 18 (9 PORTIONS)

COCONUT PYRAMIDS

4 egg yolks or two whole eggs
75 g (3 oz) caster sugar

juice and rind of half a lemon
250 g (8 oz) desiccated (dried and
shredded) coconut

Beat the egg yolks and sugar until creamy. Stir in the lemon juice, rind and coconut. Form into pyramid shapes, either with your hands or using a moist egg cup, and place on a greased baking tray. Bake at 190°C (375°F/Mark 5) until the tips are golden brown. Keep in an airtight tin or freeze. MAKES ABOUT 24 (12 PORTIONS)

GINGER CAKE WOBR

100 g (4 oz) margarine
75 g (3 oz) dark muscovado sugar
150 ml (¼ pint) golden syrup
150 ml (¼ pint) black treacle
2 tsp ground ginger
½ tsp mixed spice

½ to 1 tsp baking powder
50 g (2 oz) maize meal
100 g (4 oz) potato flour
75 g (3 oz) rice flour
150 ml (¼ pint) milk
2 eggs

Grease a 20 cm (8 in) round cake tin. Melt the margarine, sugar, syrup and treacle and stir in the spices. Sift the flour and baking powder in a bowl and make a well in the centre. Add the syrup mixture and beat until smooth. Lightly beat the eggs and milk and gradually beat into the batter. Pour into the tin and bake at 160°C (320°F/Mark 3) for one hour. Add icing if wanted. MAKES 8 GENEROUS SLICES.

LEMON AND ALMOND CAKE WOBR

175 g (6 oz) soft butter
175 g (6 oz) caster sugar
3 eggs
175 g (6 oz) self-raising flour or
brown rice flour

150 g (5 oz) ground almonds
Grated rind and juice of one lemon
½ tsp almond essence
2 lemons
2 tsp of clear honey

Pre-heat the oven to 160°C (320°F/Mark 3). Grease and base line a 20 cm (8 in) loose-bottomed round cake tin. Place the cake ingredients in a large bowl. Mix well and beat with a wooden spoon or electric whisk for 2–3 minutes until light and fluffy. Turn the mixture into the cake tin and smooth the top. Pare the rind and the pith of the two lemons, then slice into thin round slices and place on top of the cake. Bake for 50–60 minutes until golden and firm. Cool in the tin for 10 minutes then release the sides and cool on a wire rack. Warm the honey and brush over the cake. Serve immediately. SERVES 8–10.

MANGO DELIGHT WOBR

This is a delicious dessert which consists of a base of mango flesh, a custard centre and a meringue topping.

Base and custard	*Floating islands*
4 large ripe mangoes	2 large egg whites
125 g (5 oz) mascarpone cheese	4 tbsp caster sugar
125 g (5 oz) ricotta cheese	dish 12 in × 9in × 2 in.
2–3 tbsp orange juice (if necessary)	

Slice the fleshy part of the mangoes either side of the stone. Cut the mangoes into lengthways slices. Use them to line the base of a dish about 30 × 23 × 5 cm (12 × 9 × 2 in). Remove the remaining flesh from around the stone. Place it in a liquidizer in preparation for the custard. The base of the dish should be totally covered with a generous amount of the flesh of the mangoes.

Scrape the excess flesh and juice from the mango skins. Place in liquidizer with the mascarpone and ricotta cheese. If the mangoes are not sufficiently ripe, add 2–3 tbsp of orange juice and liquidize. This should produce a thick and runny custard. Cover the mangoes totally with the custard and refrigerate the dish.

Whisk the egg whites to form stiff peaks. Fold in the caster sugar. In a large baking dish add 1 cm (½ in) of cold water. Using a large spoon drop portions of the meringue on to the water. Cook in a moderate oven for 12–15 minutes until lightly brown. Take out with a slotted spoon, drain and place on top of the custard. You should have sufficient meringues to cover the whole of the dish.

CHAPTER

18

STRESS OR DISTRESS?

Let's first take a look at the terms stress and distress. In my opinion a certain amount of stress in life gets the adrenaline going and can be both mentally stimulating and healthy. When the pressure rises to the point where it then becomes uncomfortable, you can rest assured that you've hit the band of distress.

Don't ever underestimate the power of distress on your physical and mental well-being. I've seen many a 'strong' person bite the dust when under incredible pressure. The classic case is a person who seems to cope amazingly well with a disaster or a near-tragedy. They sail through the event appearing cool, calm and collected. Then several months later get physically sick or become emotionally unbalanced. It is now understood that stress places extra nutritional demands on the body. And when we are feeling stressed we often don't eat as well as usual, which can make matters worse.

Part of the game is being able to identify the source of stress and admit honestly that you are finding it a strain.

When you are feeling on top of the world physically and mentally your tolerance of problems or particularly difficult situations may be higher. Whereas when you feel below par, extra problems often seem too much to bear.

Many a physical and emotional illness is precipitated by stress. The body's demand for B vitamins increases when under stress. Often, when people have severe problems, their diet suffers and they either eat insufficient food to meet their requirements or indulge in too much junk food and alcohol. You will have seen from Chapter 14 how deficiencies in B vitamins can lead to nervous and mental disorders. Food allergies are also often linked to distressing situations. These can affect the mind and the body. Migraine headaches, irritable bowel syndrome, agoraphobia, diarrhoea, depression, insomnia, nervous tension, mood swings, restlessness, etc. can all result from stress-induced food intolerance.

A PROBLEM SHARED IS A PROBLEM HALVED

There is no need to pretend you aren't suffering: it's far better to talk over your problems and frustrations, and even have a good cry if you feel like it. Crying can be very therapeutic. Once the problem has been talked through, you may find it gets put a little more into perspective. You may suddenly realize how to cope with the situation immediately, or in the long term. Support and reassurance are very comforting: having a friend to lean on at times of great need is a very valuable asset. There is no substitute for plenty of open, honest communication.

Try to stand outside the problem and examine it carefully. This often helps you to see things more clearly. Sometimes, being so involved in a situation means you can't 'see the wood for the trees'.

Most of all, take time out each day to get your attention off the problem. Consciously daydream, if you like, in a quiet room undisturbed, or go for a long country walk and observe the wonders of nature. Discipline yourself to do this regularly. You'll be surprised how therapeutic these activities can be.

HOW STRESS AFFECTS YOUR BODY

Pay attention to your body telling you it's not very happy. Look out for possible weak areas that are more susceptible to tension build-up. For example:

Forehead	Upper back
Face	Lower back
Neck	Hands
Shoulders	Legs

Clenched teeth, grinding teeth at night, headaches and eye strain are all signs of inner stress. Becoming aware of your weaknesses is half the battle. The stresses and strains of life do tend to build up in the body. We are each affected differently. Some people suffer backaches, whilst others get headaches. When the body becomes loaded with tension we tie up our energy to some extent. The energy flows become blocked and as a result symptoms like headaches and abdominal cramps are likely to become worse. You can gently massage any tense areas or have someone do it for you, preferably each day. Also try to spend 10–15 minutes at the end of the day consciously relaxing your muscles, beginning with your face and working your way down to your toes.

A good massage is soothing. If you haven't already discovered aromatherapy oils you should try them. Lavender and geranium are two of the relaxing oils that can be used in an almond-oil base.

- Get some almond oil from the chemist and pour out a couple of tablespoons in a bowl.

- Add 12 drops of lavender or geranium aromatherapy oil.

- You can massage the bits that you can reach yourself while practising deep breathing

- or better still, get your partner or friend to give you a regular massage – it's very relaxing and generally therapeutic.

Yoga may help and it is easy to practise simple relaxing techniques at home. There are other suggestions to help you through difficult periods. Meditation, autogenic training and physical exercise seem to be beneficial for some people. It's really a question of choosing a method of relaxation which you are happy to practise regularly.

There are certain areas in your life which you might like to examine if you are feeling stressed.

- Have you taken on so many commitments that you aren't able to really enjoy life?

Some people just can't say 'No'. They have good hearts, and little appreciation of their actual working capacity. If you are guilty of this, do sit back and have a good think about it. Make yourself a work schedule and a leisure schedule and stick to it.

- Have you got any goals or aims in life you are pursuing? Having a strong sense of purpose in life is a great asset. Not having a purpose or direction can have repercussions on your mental well-being and subsequently affect your health. Without a desire to achieve something, life often becomes rather boring and meaningless.

- Have you got many unfinished projects on the go, and never seem to get around to finishing any one of them?

Knowing that you should have completed a project and didn't, especially if it's something promised to another, can be stressful. Make a list of any unfinished projects and then assign a regular time each week, to work through them gradually.

- Is your home and/or work environment tidy and in order, or have you allowed things to pile up around you?

It is difficult to thrive or relax properly in an area which is untidy, disordered or dirty. If you feel there is room for improvement, why not have a grand 'sort out' or clean up – I'll bet you feel better afterwards.

- Do you have plenty of interests and activities to pursue in your spare time? It is healthy to maintain a wide variety of interests: perhaps some activities that you like to indulge in yourself, and also activities and interests you can share with other members of your family, friends and pets.

- Do you take regular exercise and set aside relaxation time for yourself? Exercise and relaxation are both extremely valuable pursuits and contribute greatly to health. The next chapter is on the subject of exercise and should help you to work out an activity plan.

19

THE VALUE OF
EXERCISE AND
RELAXATION

I can't emphasize strongly enough how important exercise and relaxation are in maintaining a healthy body. There have been several studies which demonstrated that exercise was a valuable tool in overcoming depression, and the PMS A symptoms of nervous tension, mood swings, irritability and anxiety. And we should also bear in mind that regular exercise, particularly weight-bearing exercise, will help strengthen our bones and thus prevent the bone-thinning disease, osteoporosis, later in life.

If you don't like structural exercises you should at least take a brisk walk for half an hour a day. Personally I find swimming one of the most stimulating exercises, especially at the start of the day, or using an exercise video at home, especially on dark mornings when venturing outside may not be too appealing.

Beyond doubt, exercise raises energy levels, and your spirits. On a regular basis, it also speeds up the metabolism of the body. Although you may have to push yourself initially, I assure you it will pay dividends within a short space of time.

The mind and body work closely together. The mental stress of PMS will be reflected in the physical tension in your body. The muscular aches and pains of PMS such as headaches, neck pain and stiff joints, together with the more obvious low backache and abdominal cramps, all work to increase feelings of anxiety and depression. It's hardly surprising that the heart rate increases, as the nervous and physical tension increases, all adding to feelings of being 'wound up'.

Exercise may provide help for PMS sufferers more than just by acting as a general tonic. Several studies now show that the level of a particular brain hormone, beta-endorphin, a hormone associated with a sense of well-being and pain relief, was found to be low in pre-menstrual sufferers in the few days before their period. The levels during the first phase of the menstrual cycle were normal when compared with healthy women who did not have PMS. Beta-endorphin is an important self-produced hormone, which may affect mood and well-being, and also influence the function of other hormones. Its level can be raised by regular and usually prolonged physical exercise. Potentially, it could also be influenced by dietary and nutritional factors.

Thus, regular physical exercise by stimulating the body's natural production of beta-endorphin might help to prevent the dip that occurs premenstrually in PMS sufferers. The value of exercise in PMS has been studied in two papers from North America. Both of these report a modest benefit of aerobic exercise on PMS, especially for mental symptoms. Breast tenderness was not helped very much by this approach. My own experience supports this. Other studies have shown that physical exercise can be of value in the treatment of depression.

However, you can have too much exercise as well. Analysis of a large group of sufferers contacting the WNAS revealed that the least symptoms were experienced by those who exercised three or four times per week. Those who exercised every day had as much PMS as other women but with a smaller degree of relief in the week after their period.

GENERAL ADVICE

- It is important to take time off to care for yourself.

- Ensure that exercise and relaxation become part of your daily lifestyle.

- Choose styles of exercise that suit your personality and lifestyle.

- Make an effort to slow down at the critical time and look to ways of calming your mind and body – particularly important if your co-ordination suffers and you become clumsy.

- Above all, take a programme of exercise that balances the 3 'S's with some 'R' – universally known as:

STRENGTH, STAMINA, SUPPLENESS AND RELAXATION

Taking each of the elements in turn, I have highlighted the important factors.

S for Strength can be described as the maximum force needed by a muscle or group of muscles to overcome a resistance.

In everyday terms this means being able to push, pull, lift, climb and carry without injuring yourself. Strong back and abdominal muscles will help improve your posture and guard you from most lower back pain.

There is another important element of strength to consider and that is:

E for Endurance is the muscle's ability repeatedly to perform or maintain a task for a prolonged period of time.

There is also cardiovascular (heart and blood vessel function) training which partners muscular endurance training. Different forms of activity will improve the endurance qualities of different muscle groups. For example, running will train the leg muscles much more than the upper body and arms, while swimming will emphasize upper body endurance. Both, however, will increase cardiovascular endurance.

S for Stamina simply means being able to keep going; whether you're walking, swimming, running or cycling – and without stopping or becoming tired!

These types of activity are called 'aerobic' because of the increased need for oxygen by the working muscles. Remember, the heart is a muscle too and it needs exercise just as much as your legs or arms. The lungs are used to oxygenate the blood. With regular exercise, the heart and lungs become more efficient. The benefits of aerobic training mean you eventually achieve better results with less effort. Your heart and lungs will have to work less hard in daily life.

Experts disagree as to exactly how much aerobic exercise you need to benefit or gain from the training effect. It will also vary from person to person. A general rule of thumb is to aim for at least 20 minutes about three times a week.

S for Suppleness and flexibility: the ability to move your joints through their full range of movement. In other words, being able to bend, stretch, reach and turn to your fullest. Of all the fitness elements so far, flexibility must rate as the one most likely to affect your everyday life. It also means protecting your muscles and joints from injury and stiffness, as well as improving your circulation, posture and poise.

Improving your range of movement will also help to improve your performance in other activities. Correct stretching, when practised after your exercise session (as well as before), will help to minimize the likelihood of post-exercise soreness.

R for Relaxation is the art of letting go. Knowing how to let go and with confidence, is probably one of the most important elements of health and fitness. The ability to release unnecessary muscular tension and calm the mind is a wonderful resource to call upon. Tension is tiring and unproductive.

For some, exercise itself is a form of relaxation, while others might turn to a hobby or pastime.

Relaxation and breathing go hand in hand. Indeed, improving your breathing patterns during exercise is one of the keys to success. It also engenders a feeling of alertness and readiness to cope.

Over the weeks of a considered programme of exercise you will increase the efficiency of your heart and lung capacity with deeper breathing.

TIPS AND HINTS ON EXERCISING

To really ensure you gain the maximum benefit from your efforts, take a few moments to read the following tips and hints – they make all the difference to how you feel about your exercising.

- Remember, exercise should be fun and something you look forward to.

- It won't be if you push yourself fast and furiously, it will only leave you exhausted, sore and disappointed with your efforts.

- Really listen to your body. Believe it or not, it knows best!

- Take it slowly and gradually for longer-lasting results.

- Take time to work out your fitness aims and objectives – what do you want to achieve from your efforts? Finding and following the right programme for you is as vital as eating the right food.

- Decide which activity, or blend of activities, will suit you and help to realize your aims.

- Mix and match whenever possible. Avoid boredom by choosing from several activities you know that you will enjoy and stick at. Better still, are they convenient and can you enjoy the company of others at the same time?

- Try to combine some of your exercises with fresh air and sunlight, both of which have proven benefit in helping to relieve PMS symptoms.

- Balance is the key to successful exercising. Give upper and lower body the same amount of work and spread the load.

- Don't expect miracles overnight – be patient and persevere!

- Aim for quality of exercise, not quantity – look forward to it and enjoy it.

PRECAUTIONS

Most people do not need a full medical check-up before exercising, but if you answer YES to any of the following questions, or you are over 35 and a 'first timer', it's best to discuss your plans with your doctor.

Have you ever suffered from, or is there a family history of:

Chest pains or pain in the shoulders?
High blood pressure or heart disease?
Chest problems like asthma or bronchitis?
Back pain or joint pains?
Headaches, faintness or feelings of nausea?
Diabetes?
Are you taking any medication?
Are you recovering from illness or recent operations?
Are you very overweight?
Are you pregnant?

If you have a cold or sore throat, give exercise a miss until you feel better. When you do resume, take it slowly and build up to your pre-illness fitness level gradually. If you ever feel pain, dizziness, nausea or undue tiredness whenever or wherever you exercise, STOP immediately. Rest and wait. Change your position or slacken off the intensity if relevant. Try again. If the complaint persists, stop and seek professional advice.

Posture pointers

- Stand in front of a full-length mirror with feet about hip-width apart and insteps lifted.

- Gently rock back and forth to find your balance and 'centred' position. Body-weight will feel evenly balanced between balls and heels, as well as inner and outer edges of feet.

- Line knees directly over ankles and gently pull up thigh muscles above the knees.

The standing position

Now stand sideways to the mirror. Push your bottom out and see and feel the lower back arch and tummy bulge. Correct this by pulling in the abdominal muscles and tucking the buttocks under you. See and feel the lower back lengthen as the pubic bone (pelvis) tilts up to the ceiling. This is the pelvic tilt.

- Keep hips level and maintain pelvic tilt as you turn to face mirror.

- Lift ribcage up and away from hips.

- Pull shoulders down from ears; keep them level and aligned over ankles.

- Let arms hang loosely.

- Lift head upwards from crown and feel the back of neck lengthen.

- Hold chin at right angle to ground.

- Feel entire spine lengthen.

Run through these posture pointers and the pelvic tilt frequently throughout the day, to maintain alignment and heighten your awareness.

Warm-up

Now you're ready to warm up. Never miss out this section as it prepares your body for the work to follow. Mobilizing and loosening exercises, plus some preliminary stretches, will help to improve your performance and skill by increasing the body temperature. A warm-up also helps to reduce the risk of injury and soreness. About 10 minutes is all most people need. Similarly, 'warm down' at the end of each session – no matter how rushed you are. End with some rhythmical exercises and slow holding stretches that taper down from more demanding ones. A warm-down will induce a feeling of relaxation and well-being. It will also help to reduce the likelihood of post-exercise stiffness and soreness.

Warm up by moving rhythmically for 10 minutes to your favourite piece of music, working from your feet upwards, gradually using your whole body.

During your warm-down, take it easy, hold your stretches and slow down gradually. This will minimize any soreness and stiffness.

Relieve the tension

This section takes a look at specific exercises and steps you can take to release tension associated with PMS, as well as improve posture and awareness.

Deeper breathing will be promoted, as well as relaxation and a feeling of calm.

Shoulders and neck

Tension and tightness generally collect at the base of the neck and across tops of shoulders. They are mostly due to the way we sit and stand, as well as being our natural reaction to stress – we slouch, so the neck collapses and the shoulders hunch. Not a pretty sight and often it leaves us with a headache due to the constriction of blood supply to and from the brain.

Take positive steps to ovecome these problems by loosening shoulders and paying more attention to posture. See posture pointers on page 238.

To start, stand or sit well with the head centred and breathe well as you:

1. Lift both shoulders up, pull them back and strongly down. Repeat several times.

Tip – Make sure you really squeeze into the upper back and keep chin held in.

2. Clasp hands loosely behind lower back and rest them just above buttocks.

Keep elbows bent and hands resting on body throughout.

Squeeze between the shoulder blades so the elbows draw together.

Hold and release slowly.

Repeat several times.

Feel the squeeze between the shoulder blades and the stretch across the chest.

Tip – Keep the shoulders down, head centred and lower back straight.

3. Turn head slowly to look over right shoulder while maintaining length in the neck and keeping shoulders still.

Return to centre and repeat to opposite side.

Repeat several times.

Return to centre and pull chin in to lengthen back of neck.

Tilt head slowly to right shoulder while keeping shoulders level.

Feel the stretch on the opposite side.

Return slowly to centre.

Tip – As you tilt head, imagine you are looking into a mirror to see both cheeks evenly.

Finally, return to centre, pull shoulders down and tuck chin in.

Tilt head gently forwards.

Feel the stretch along the neck.

Return to centre and repeat once more, breathing well.

Back and hips

1. Back strengthener

Lie on your front on either a mat or rug, with legs together, forehead on floor and chin tucked in.

Clasp hands loosely and rest them on lower back.

As you breathe out, contract abdominal and buttock muscles and squeeze between the shoulder blades.

Straighten arms down towards your feet and raise chest, shoulders and forehead off the floor to form one continuous line.

Lower slowly to the floor and repeat once more.

2. Back release

From the previous exercise, place hands under shoulders and gently push up on to your knees to lower your bottom back on to your heels.

Fold your body forwards to rest chest on thighs.

Tuck your head down and rest arms down by sides of body.

Tip – If you feel claustrophobic, stretch your arms out in front of you and rest forehead lightly on floor.

3. Pelvic tilt

Use the pelvic tilt as a back release as well as a preliminary movement to abdominal strengtheners.

Pelvic tilts can be done standing, sitting or lying. Take time to practise the movement, as getting it right makes all the difference to the safety and effectiveness of your exercising and alignment.

Start by lying back on a mat or rug.

Bend knees with feet hip-width apart and lengthen back of neck by tucking chin in.

As you breathe out, press lower back down on to mat and pull in abdominal muscles.

Feel the pubic bone tilt up to the ceiling and the lower back flatten down against the floor.

Practise several times until you feel confident of the movement.

4. Curl-overs to strengthen abdominal muscles

Strong abdominal muscles help prevent some lower back pain.

Start as for the pelvic tilt and rest hands on your thighs.

As you breathe out, pelvic tilt and curl head and shoulders slowly off the floor, sliding hands towards knees.

Hold for count of four with waist and lower back on floor.

Lie back slowly and repeat four times.

Let go!

Having the ability to release tension and calm the mind is a wonderful resource to call upon. Tension is tiring and wasteful. Knowing how to cope and apply positive resources is the key to successful relaxation. Adopt any position you find comfortable and supportive for your lower back and neck. It may mean sitting in a high-back chair, or lying back with neck supported by a cushion and legs resting on a chair or stool.

Use your breathing to enhance your relaxation and let your restorative side take over.

Remember to pull the shoulders well down from the ears and let arms rest heavily.

Take several deep breaths, feeling the ribcage move up and out like bellows as you breathe in, and downwards as you breathe out.

Your breathing will gradually become more rhythmical as you start to let go.

Run down your body and check where you feel tight.

Are your shoulders up round your ears? Pull them down. Are your hands clenched? Stretch them out and let the fingers curl.

What about your buttocks and lower back? Make an extra effort to relax and release – try the pelvic tilt to prevent back aching.

Concentrate on your legs, particularly ankles and feet. Let them go and feel the whole body soften.

Finally pay attention to your mouth and face. Soften the jaw and let the softness spread over your face – around the nostrils, between and over your eyes and across your forehead to your hairline.

Spend a few quiet moments with yourself.

When you feel ready, take a few deep breaths, have a good stretch and yawn before curling over to one side and sitting up slowly.

20

OTHER VALUABLE
THERAPIES

As well as dealing with symptoms on a nutritional level it is important to make sure that your whole body is functioning at optimum level. The years during which you may have suffered nutritional deficiencies, while coping with stressful situations and pre-menstrual symptoms, may well have taken their toll. The body is a very complicated, but delicate network of bones, muscles, ligaments, nerves, organs and blood vessels. Physical symptoms and nervous tension can affect the smooth running of the body processes. When you make a start on your nutritional programme, if your symptoms are intense, you might consider the value of cranial osteopathy, acupuncture, or acupressure. They are powerful tools and can help to bring about speedy relief of symptoms.

OSTEOPATHY

It is not uncommon, through the wear and tear of everyday life, for subtle back or neck problems to occur. I have seen many resistant, long-standing headaches cured by some good osteopathic manipulation. It is certainly worth having a check-up with a qualified osteopath if you feel tension building up in your back or neck, or if you suffer regular headaches.

Cranial osteopathy, or cranio-sacral therapy as it is known, is a specialized form of osteopathy. Unlike conventional osteopathy, it is a gentle yet potent form of therapy. The aim is gently to coax the muscles, tendons, joints and connective tissue to establish correct functions and release restrictions, thus restoring normal circulation, flow of energy and glandular secretions.

The cranio-sacral mechanism is comprised of the cranium (the skull), the sacrum (the bone at the base of the spine), the membranes surrounding the brain, the spinal cord and the fascia of continuous, clingfilm-like sheet that surrounds the muscles, organs, joints and bones. The tension of this fascia, the clingfilm-like lining, is all important. If you have ever worn an all-in-one pants suit that is too tight or too short in the body, you will have experienced some discomfort. If the tension in the body's fascia becomes too tight, you can't just take it off like an uncomfortable piece of clothing, and it is possible that body functions can be affected in the long term.

Cranial osteopaths claim a good success rate with women who have PMS and other menstrual disorders. You will find it very gentle treatment. Here are some experiences of a cranial osteopath who regularly treats women with PMS and menstrual problems. As well as her treatment she recommends that her patients take regular exercise and seek nutritional advice.

Case history 1

The patient experienced migraine and PMS for five to six days prior to each period. She had some lower back strain, reduced mobility in her upper neck and some pelvic congestion. Her neck was treated and normal function restored. As a result, the congestion and strain within the skull were reduced, the migraines were instantly alleviated, and the PMS symptoms reduced. The patient then received nutritional advice and her PMS reduced further.

Case history 2

This patient was a woman aged 44 who suffered with severe PMS, and backache before and during her period. She was very tall and had poor posture. When examined, she had restricted movement in the lower back and pelvic congestion. After treatment over a period of two months she became 90 per cent better.

It is certainly worth finding a local practitioner if you feel the need is there. (See page 276.)

ACUPUNCTURE AND ACUPRESSURE

It is worth mentioning the contribution made by traditional Chinese medicine in the treatment of female health problems. According to the severity of the problem, there are two levels at which treatment can be taken. The first level is appropriate for severe symptoms and involves consulting an acupuncturist. Many of the problems mentioned, including PMS, painful periods, irregular periods, fluid retention and distension, pelvic inflammation, migraines, backache, morning sickness and other troubles of pregnancy, menopausal symptoms, depression, anxiety and insomnia may all respond to treatment by acupuncture. If you feel your complaint is too serious or persistent to cope with by yourself, acupuncture is worth considering as a possible option.

Of course you should always ensure that you get help from a properly trained and registered practitioner. You can usually obtain information from your public library or Citizens Advice Bureau. A register is published by the Council for Acupuncture, listing all members of the four recognized and affiliated professional bodies.

As we are concentrating on aspects of self-help, it is worth considering a second level of treatment, more appropriate to the minor or occasional problems which you can sometimes alleviate by self-assessment and treatment at home. This can be done through Shiatsu, the Japanese finger pressure method (sometimes called acupressure). In this system the body is influenced in various ways by stimulating key points, found along the course of energy channels circulating near the skin surface. These are the same as acupuncture meridians, but the points are stimulated by pressure rather than needles.

For Shiatsu to be effective it is important to give the right kind of pressure, for an appropriate length of time. It is no good pushing pressure points like 'magic buttons' and it is important to recognize by the feel whether what you are doing is correct. Provided you adopt the right approach, Shiatsu may be very helpful, whether you enlist the help of a friend or perform it on your own (self-Shiatsu).

Here is a summary of the method and a description of how to find just a few of the most useful points for some of the troubles mentioned.

Pre-menstrual depression/anxiety

First, try working along the inner leg. Also, two inches above the wrist, in between the tendons at the centre of the inner arm, there is a good point to press firmly. Breathing is very important to get your energy flowing smoothly, so try this simple exercise. Kneel on a cushion or carpeted floor and join your hands together with the fingers back to back while pointing the fingertips towards your own upper abdomen. Let your relaxed fingers press into the centre, below the ribs but above the navel. As you do this lean gently forward and exhale. The pressure should lend a little force to the exhalation. Wait for the inhalation to come naturally and raise yourself back again to the upright kneeling position while breathing in. Go gently at first, repeating the action with every breath, leaning a bit further on to your fingers each time. The abdominal muscles may seem tight or tender but try to relax fully at the end of each breath while leaning forward. Only do this 10 times. You may move your fingers up and down or a little way along the ribs to explore for any tension. Afterwards sit quietly for a minute. You may feel like a good stretch before getting up.

Insomnia/headaches

Work with your own fingertips along the base of the skull behind the head where it joins the neck. Feel for any sensitive hollows where the muscles meet the bony ridge and, leaning your head back, let your fingers penetrate and hold for a few breaths. (If you do this for a friend, support her forehead with one hand and use your other hand to find points with finger and thumb on either side of her neck, pressing inward and upward.) For frontal headaches lean forward, letting your fingertips support the forehead just below the eyebrows – it may feel tender, but breathe and relax for several seconds. Also, work generally along the inside edges and soles of the feet, pressing especially around the inside ankle area. Another useful point for headaches can be found by pressing hard into the fleshy area between your finger and thumb – press towards the edge of the bone on the forefinger side.

Period pains

Get comfortable. Feel for sensitive points along the inside of the lower leg between the edge of the bone and the calf muscle. Hold any points with sustained thumb-pressure to the limit of comfort for five or six seconds or longer. You should try to breathe easily in a relaxed way and maintain the pressure until the sensation diminishes a little. To make it easier, reinforce one thumb with the other while pressing. Ask a friend or partner to lean with their thumbs into the area of the sacrum (triangular bony part at the base of your spine between the buttocks), they could explore a little way each side of centre, pressing firmly but gently any tender spots they find (you should say if it is too strong).

If this approach really interests you, there are two particularly good books you could read which are mentioned on the Reading List on page 274. You could also look for Shiatsu classes in your area. If you do not know of any, write to the secretary of the Shiatsu Society whose address is listed in Appendix 5 at the back of the book, page 278. The Society will send you a list of qualified teachers.

Whatever you do, it is important to ensure that you put yourself in the hands of a qualified practitioner. These days all the recognized alternative therapies have official associations. These bodies keep registers of qualified practitioners. It is best to check up as there are, sadly, quite a few non-qualified practitioners who are not to be recommended.

21

OTHER
RELATED PROBLEMS

By now you should have a good idea of what may be causing your pre-
menstrual symptoms and how you can treat them successfully by changing
your diet, taking some nutritional supplements and doing some moderate
exercise. Very often PMS exists together with other health problems. This
may be by chance, but sometimes there is a dietary connection. In this
chapter I want to take a brief look at some common health problems and
situations that sometimes occur alongside PMS or generally affect us as
women.

PAINFUL PERIODS

Painful periods are particularly common in young women, especially
before they start child-bearing but older women may sometimes
experience them as well. Period pains are not actually part of PMS and
anyone who experiences severe pain should check with their doctor and
perhaps be referred for a gynaecological check-up to see if there may be an
underlying problem.

WHAT CAUSES THEM

Period pain, referred to by doctors as dysmenorrhoea, most often occurs
because of excessive muscle contractions of the uterus with each period.

There are four common gynaecological problems which may cause the periods to become painful. These include:

- infection of the tubes or ovaries

- fibroids

- endometriosis, where the lining of the womb is found in other tissues such as the wall of the uterus or around the ovaries

- a deficiency of the mineral magnesium, the most commonly deficient nutrient in women of child-bearing age, which is needed for optimum muscle function.

Often, however, there is no problem with the anatomy. Periods can continue to be painful for the first 24 to 48 hours and perhaps even the day before the period begins. Period pain is often felt as mild to severe cramp-like pains or discomfort in the lower abdomen. It can also be felt as low back pain or aching down the legs and, when severe, can be accompanied by giddiness, faintness, nausea and even occasional vomiting. These other symptoms are probably due to the hormonal and chemical changes that occur at the time of the period.

There are a variety of treatments that exist that may be helpful, some of which can be administered by your doctor and others which you can undertake as self-help measures.

- **Magnesium check** Measure your red cell magnesium, to see whether you have a deficiency. This is a simple blood test and should be readily available.

- **Painkillers** Your doctor may recommend the use of certain types of painkillers or hormonal products. Some mild painkillers may not be very effective for severe pain but a more powerful sort which are either prescribable (mefenamic acid-Ponstan) or available on the advice of your pharmacist can be particularly useful. It may be necessary to try a number before finding the most effective one for you.

- **The contraceptive pill** A number of hormonal preparations are available but often the most useful, particularly in young women who require contraception, is the oral contraceptive pill. The most modern low dose pills have much fewer side-effects than older preparations.

- **Iron** Your doctor can prescribe iron supplements if you are anaemic as well.

The self-help measures include:

- Taking regular physical exercise which may be helpful with a variety of period-related problems and may help improve your tolerance of pain. Aim to exercise three or four times a week, and during a painful period try to do some gentle yoga exercises or relaxation instead of strenuous exercise.

- Eat a diet rich in essential fatty acids, especially fish oils (see page 163). Women with period pains are known to have lower intakes of these oils, which may have anti-inflammatory and painkilling properties.

- Some minerals may also be helpful. Magnesium is particularly important in muscle and hormonal functions. It balances with calcium and influences the contraction of the muscles of the uterus. One study suggests that it may help to reduce period pain. Good dietary sources of magnesium can be found on page 161.

- Improving your diet can also help to correct hormonal abnormalities, some of which are thought to underlie gynaecological problems. Cut down on fatty food and have a good intake of fibre from fruit and vegetables which may help to control hormone metabolism and reduce some of the excessive hormone swings that occur during the menstrual cycle.

- Heat seems to have a soothing effect on muscles. Apply a hot water bottle or thermal heat pad to your tummy to help ease the pain.

- Both acupuncture and cranial osteopathy may help to free up pockets of blocked energy in the body. Herbal and homoeopathic remedies are also worth a try. If the pain is caused by an infection, this will need to be dealt with by conventional medicine; however, complementary therapy will also help to boost the immune system which increases your resistence to infection in the long term.

Magnesium supplements can be obtained from healthfood shops. At the WNAS we tend to use magnesium amino acid chelate to what we call 'gut tolerance' level. In other words, if you take too much you will get diarrhoea. A magnesium-rich multi-mineral supplement may also be helpful.

Heat is helpful, too, as it helps to relax the muscles. Placing a heat pad inside your clothes or taking a hot water bottle to bed can be very soothing.

If these self-help measures do not reduce your pain considerably it is wise to consult your general practitioner or family planning clinic.

Often when nutritional supplements have been corrected particularly low magnesium levels, and the muscles are functioning normally, period pains subside. It may therefore be worth following this self-help advice for a few months before seeking further advice.

HEAVY PERIODS

Excessive loss of blood is a problem for up to 10 per cent of menstruating women and is the main factor that leads to iron deficiency and anaemia in women of child-bearing age. On average, we lose just over 2 tablespoons (35 ml) of blood during a period and a heavy period, or menorrhagia as it is technically known, constitutes 5 tablespoons (80 ml) which is considerably more than average. It is hard to assess the precise loss during a period. Even scientific studies to assess the numbers of towels or tampons we use through a period were inaccurate, as it seems that women change their sanitary protection after collecting differing amounts of blood.

Periods tend to get a little heavier with increasing age and with increasing weight but there are other factors too. The possible underlying causes include:

- An early miscarriage. Sometimes a woman may conceive without realizing, but because it is an unviable pregnancy Mother Nature terminates it, in the form of what appears to be a very heavy period.

- A hormonal imbalance in the body.

- A recently fitted IUD can result in heavy periods, which usually settle down after the first few months.

- The presence of fibroids in the uterus can increase the flow of a period.

- Approaching the menopause, the lining of the uterus can become thicker, resulting in heavier blood loss.

- In our experience heavy periods can be caused sometimes by nutritional deficiencies.

If your periods become unmanageably heavy, or you have a sudden episode of flooding, you should consult your doctor for advice. After taking a history of the problem, your doctor will:

- Take some blood for a serum ferritin test to check whether your iron stores are in fact low, in which case you would need a course of iron.

- Examine you to determine whether there are any fibroids present or any other physical abnormalities, in which case you would then be referred to a gynaecologist who would decide whether you need minor surgery.

- Remove your IUD if you have one, to see whether that alters the flow.

- Prescribe transexamic acid, a drug that helps excessive bleeding. It can be more effective than hormones.

- Prescribe hormone pills to reduce the flow. The first choice for a younger woman might be the oral contraceptive pill; failing that, Duphaston, a progestogen preparation; and if that fails to work, then Danazol, which has considerable side-effects.

- Doctors sometimes suggest a hysterectomy which should be regarded as a last resort. If you do decide to part with your uterus think very carefully before having your ovaries removed. (See Every Woman's Health Guide, page 275.)

The self-help measures that you can implement are to:

- Take a good, strong multi-vitamin and mineral supplements with extra B vitamins, vitamin C with bioflavinoids and magnesium.

- Eat plenty of green leafy vegetables, liver, free-range eggs and other foods rich in iron.

- Rest when the flow is heavy and avoid important social engagements until the bleeding has reduced.

- Consult a herbal practitioner or a homoeopath for a remedy to fit your individual symptoms.

SONIA

SYMPTOMS

	WEEK AFTER PERIOD (Fill in 3 days after period)				WEEK BEFORE PERIOD (Fill in 2-3 days before period)			
	None	Mild	Moderate	Severe	None	Mild	Moderate	Severe
PMS - A								
Nervous Tension	✓						✓	
Mood Swings	✓							✓
Irritability	✓							✓
Anxiety	✓						✓	
PMS - H								
*Weight Gain	✓						✓	
Swelling of Extremities	✓				✓			
Breast Tenderness	✓						✓	
Abdominal Bloating	✓					✓		
PMS - C								
Headache	✓					✓		
Craving for Sweets	✓							✓
Increased Appetite	✓						✓	
Heart Pounding	✓				✓			
Fatigue		✓					✓	
Dizziness or Fainting	✓					✓		
PMS - D								
Depression		✓					✓	
Forgetfulness		✓					✓	
Crying	✓					✓		
Confusion	✓						✓	
Insomnia	✓				✓			
OTHER SYMPTOMS								
Loss of Sexual Interest	✓					✓		
Disorientation	✓				✓			
Clumsiness							✓	
Tremors/Shakes	✓				✓			
Thoughts of Suicide	✓				✓			
Agoraphobia	✓				✓			
Increased Physical Activity	✓				✓			
Heavy/Aching Legs	✓					✓		
Generalized Aches	✓					✓		
Bad Breath	✓				✓			
Sensitivity to Music/Light	✓				✓			
Excessive Thirst		✓				✓		

Do you have any other PRE-MENSTRUAL SYMPTOMS not listed above?

1. _____

2. _____

3. _____

4. _____

*5. How much weight do you gain before your period? __4 lbs approx__

254

FOLLOW UP
PRE-MENSTRUAL SYNDROME QUESTIONNAIRE

Name: Sonia   Age: 39   Height: 5' 1"   Weight: 8st 8lb

MARITAL STATUS: Single ✓   Married ✓   Divorced ✓   Widowed _____

(Please tick where applicable)

PRESENT CONTRACEPTION: None _____   Pill _____   I.U.D _____   Other _____

Your periods come every __28__ days   Your periods last __5-7__ days

Your periods are: Light _____   Moderate ✓   Heavy ✓

SYMPTOMS	WEEK AFTER PERIOD (Fill in 3 days after period)				WEEK BEFORE PERIOD (Fill in 2-3 days before period)			
	None	Mild	Moderate	Severe	None	Mild	Moderate	Severe
PMS - A								
Nervous Tension	✓				✓			
Mood Swings	✓				✓			
Irritability	✓				✓			
Anxiety	✓				✓			
PMS - H								
*Weight Gain	✓				✓			
Swelling of Extremities	✓				✓			
Breast Tenderness	✓					✓		
Abdominal Bloating	✓					✓		
PMS - C								
Headache	✓				✓			
Craving for Sweets	✓				✓			
Increased Appetite	✓				✓			
Heart Pounding	✓				✓			
Fatigue	✓				✓			
Dizziness or Fainting	✓				✓			
PMS - D								
Depression	✓				✓			
Forgetfulness	✓				✓			
Crying	✓				✓			
Confusion	✓				✓			
Insomnia	✓				✓			
OTHER SYMPTOMS								
Loss of Sexual Interest	✓				✓			
Disorientation	✓				✓			
Clumsiness	✓				✓			
Tremors/Shakes	✓				✓			
Thoughts of Suicide	✓				✓			
Agoraphobia	✓				✓			
Increased Physical Activity	✓				✓			
Heavy/Aching Legs	✓				✓			
Generalized Aches	✓				✓			
Bad Breath	✓				✓			
Sensitivity to Music/Light	✓				✓			
Excessive Thirst	✓				✓			

IRREGULAR OR ABSENT PERIODS

As women we were designed to have regular periods and anything between 23 and 35 days is considered to be a normal cycle length which ends with a period essentially marking a 'failed conception'. After the first year, periods usually establish a regular pattern, which becomes the normal cycle for an individual and usually continues until the menopause is approaching. Irregular periods and the absence of periods altogether often signify that eggs are not being released in the normal fashion, mid-cycle. The absence of periods is categorized by the medical profession in two ways and is referred to as amenorrhoea. Primary amenorrhoea is when no period ever arrives which is rare, and usually associated with late puberty or a defect in the hormone and reproductive system. Unfortunately, there is little that can be done to correct it. Secondary amenorrhoea is when periods have 'disappeared' for more than four cycles and there are many underlying causes, most of which can be addressed.

Periods can become irregular or disappear for a variety of reasons including pregnancy and breast feeding but in these cases it is perfectly normal. Other factors that contribute to the disruption of the menstrual cycle include:

- Anaemia and monitored deficiencies, especially of vitamin B

- Long-term medication

- Undetected and therefore untreated thyroid disease

- Episodes of extreme stress such as bereavement or divorce

- Sudden weight loss due to any illness including the slimmers' disease, anorexia nervosa

- Over-exercising which results in decreased oestrogen levels and greatly increases the chances of developing osteoporosis later in life – a problem that many ballet dancers often face.

If periods have not arrived by the age of 16 or 17 it is advisable to discuss the situation with your doctor and perhaps be referred to an endocrinologist who specialises in hormonal problems. If an established cycle has been disrupted or has disappeared then there are a number of things that can be done. First of all, your doctor can check to see whether you are pregnant which is probably the commonest reason why periods cease! Additionally, your doctor can:

- Take a blood sample to check your thyroid and iron level.

- Assess the function of your pituitary gland which is responsible for hormone function.

- If you are taking prescribed drugs, check to see whether the medication may be interrupting your cycle.

- Refer you for a gynaecological check-up to see whether your ovaries are functioning and whether there are any other underlying problems.

There are plenty of things that you can do for yourself to help restore your cycle.

- Eat wholesome food regularly by following the menus outlined in this book. You will be meeting your body's needs. Don't forget to have mid-morning and mid-afternoon snacks in your pre-menstrual week as this is when your calorie requirements are increased.

- Take regular vitamin and mineral supplements (see page 205 for suggestions).

- If you are a professional dancer, athlete or exercise addict make sure that you are meeting your calorie requirements.

- If your weight is low for your height and framework increase your weight and get some help with sorting out any stressful situations that you face, and have some counselling if you have been bereaved or recently separated or divorced.

- It may well be worth having some acupuncture which is aimed at unblocking energy channels in the body, or

- Consult a qualified homeopath or medical herbalist.

PREGNANCY

This is still the best treatment for PMS! But, alas, is not the solution. However, a sound nutritional state during pregnancy is of paramount importance, and it therefore deserves a mention, especially as some 40 per cent of pregnancies in the Western world are unplanned.

Research shows quite clearly that we can 'programme' the health of a baby and influence its growth and development, at least four months before it is even conceived, and certainly during the first three to four months of pregnancy. Our diet, environment and lifestyle can affect the shape and size of the baby and the health of its important little organs, not to mention its intelligence in later life. We can even influence the diseases this new individual will suffer in later life and its lifespan.

From the time of conception, each minute bodily system has its own timetable for development, and the supply of essential nutrients and timing of contact with a toxin would determine the type of damage that results. Babies who are undernourished in the first four weeks of development stand a much higher chance of developing heart disease, a major cause of death in middle age, and brain disorders present from birth which show up later in life in one in eight adults.

Since December 1992, the recommendation of the Chief Medical Officer for the Department of Health in the United Kingdom has been that all women who are intending to become pregnant, or who are likely to, should eat healthy diets before they conceive and take supplements that contain 400 mg of folic acid, preferably together with other B vitamins which help guard against the risk of spina bifida, other damage to the brain and nervous system. It is now acknowledged that it is difficult for a prospective mother to consume enough folic acid from her diet alone.

There are other nutrients that play an important role in the health and well-being of an infant.

- Zinc deficiency during pregnancy has been linked with low birth weight, under 2.5 kg (6 lb).

- Essential fatty acids (EFAs) are vital for growth and development of the baby, particularly for the brain and the central nervous system. Recent research suggests that a deficiency of these long-chain polyunsaturated fatty acids in the tissues of growing babies results in low birth weight, which may have life-long implications. We now know too that adequate intakes of EFAs in the new-born infant seem to influence vision and subsequent intelligence.

Babies born after an apparently normal pregnancy often have borderline levels of EFAs, as do premature babies. Breast milk from a well-nourished mother is a good source of EFAs, which probably explains why some breast-fed infants make better progress than bottle-fed ones. Trials feeding Efamarine – a combination of evening primrose and marine fish oils – to pregnant women during the final three months of pregnancy are under way. Good sources of essential fatty acids can be found on page 163 and supplements of Efanatal, designed to be taken during pregnancy, are now available from chemists and healthfood shops.

Vitamin A is another nutrient linked to growth and it has long been recommended by the Department of Health in the UK that all pregnant and breast-feeding mothers take supplements of vitamin A as beta-carotene, the non-animal source, as well as vitamins D and C, in order to build up vitamin stores that can be passed aacross the placenta. We are now, however, discouraged from eating vitamin A as retinol or to eat liver which may contain particularly large amounts of this nutrient as an excess of vitamin A as retinol is associated with congenital birth defects. If you happen to become pregnant whilst you are following the recommendations for PMS it will be necessary for you to cut the dosage of your supplements down to no more than one multi-vitamin, multi-mineral per day and to discontinue cod liver oil if you have been taking it.

So much wonderful research has been done into the area of preconception and pregnancy it is impossible to summarize it in such a short space. If there is a vague possibility that you may become pregnant, you owe it to your unborn child to consider these findings which will undoubtedly have a positive effect on the health of your baby in the long term. There are a few good books that address this area including my own which is called *Healthy Parents, Healthy Baby*. For further details see page 275.

POST-NATAL DEPRESSION

This type of depression is often referred to as the baby blues as it arrives shortly after the birth of a new baby. Symptoms vary from feeling tearful and anxious, through to a fully blown psychotic disorder which results in total rejection of the baby.

Symptoms include mood changes that vary from depression to elation, crying, insomnia, irritability and in severe cases, thoughts of suicide or actually harming the baby.

The association between depression after childbirth and pre-menstrual problems has been known for many years and was used as evidence that both conditions were due to a lack of the hormone progesterone. This has not been proved to be the case in PMS and it is a source of ongoing debate amongst the medical fraternity. There is evidence that both conditions reflect a vulnerability of the body to hormonal changes and the ability to tolerate this may, in turn, be due to both nutritional and social factors.

Post-natal depression undoubtedly needs medical supervision. Your doctor should start by checking your thyroid function including a check for thyroid antibodies, and checking your iron levels by checking your serum ferritin, and in an ideal world your levels of calcium, vitamin B6 and magnesium, all of which have been shown to be low in some women with post-natal depression.

Counselling should be on offer from your GP practice which will help you talk through your emotions when symptoms persist. Anti-depressants may be prescribed in extreme cases of post-natal depression. Help from a psychiatrist and hospital treatment may also be necessary.

A healthy diet, vitamin and mineral supplements, plenty of rest, adequate sleep and a supporting and loving environment seem to be good treatments for most cases of post-natal depression. It is noteworthy that during pregnancy and whilst breast-feeding, the demands for calcium, magnesium and B vitamins are very high, and a loss of most of these can cause changes in mood. Off-loading any responsibilities you can in the first few weeks after having a baby may help as well as taking regular exercise, preferably in the fresh air. It is often that simple.

STERILIZATION

Female sterilization is most often achieved by cutting or clipping the Fallopian tubes that normally carry the eggs released from the ovary to the womb. By preventing the union between the egg and the sperm a high degree of protection against pregnancy is achieved. The operation, known as tubal ligation, which is usually performed under general anaesthetic, can cause a few minor changes in hormone balance but these usually settle down within six months. Though it is not officially recognized as being a factor in the production of PMS, my experience is that for many women who have consulted us it appears to be an important and unwelcome influence as borne out by Jane's testimony.

> 'Ever since I was sterilized I had PMS symptoms. I never had any kind of PMS or period problems before. I went back to the doctor who sterilized me when I started to get these symptoms every month. He just turned around and said, "You women are all the same. You don't want any more babies, we sterilize you and then you come back and complain."
>
> The doctor assured me that sterilization had nothing to do with the symptoms I was getting now, but I insisted that before the sterilization I had felt perfectly OK, terrific every month and did not have any PMS symptoms whatsoever. I was very annoyed by his reaction.'

Why symptoms suddenly arrive is not really understood, although it is believed progesterone levels drop for a while after sterilization. From our experience it appears that the surgical intervention of sterilization seems to tip the hormonal scale which until the operation has been finely balanced. However, we have managed to eliminate the symptoms once again with the nutritional programme. Obviously, much more research is needed into the whole issue of the implications of nutritional deficiencies.

THE MENOPAUSE

For most women, PMS should be diminishing at the time of the menopause. This is certainly true for many, as numerous surveys have shown that the peak age for experiencing PMS symptoms is mid-thirties with a fall off thereafter. However, for some women PMS symptoms may worsen as the menopause approaches, and the two can blend together. The symptoms are quite different. At the menopause, which is characterized by the cessation of periods, there are symptoms of oestrogen deficiency such as vaginal dryness and shrinkage of breast tissue. The hot flushes and sweats are due to surges of other hormones from the pituitary gland at the base of the brain which is trying to persuade the failing ovaries to carry on working. Again, as in menstruation itself or post-delivery, there is considerable variation in individual women's ability to tolerate these hormonal changes.

The word menopause actually only refers to the time at which the last natural period takes place. It is a date rather than a period of time. Women often experience changes for as long as five years leading up to the menopause and this time is referred to as the peri-menopause. Some unfortunate women find that their Pre-Menstrual Syndrome persists as they enter the peri-menopause. In our own surveys we have looked at the relationship between previous PMS suffering and current menopausal symptoms. We found there did seem to be a moderate connection between the severity of past PMS symptoms and some current menopause symptoms, particularly symptoms of depression, anxiety, confusion and insomnia; whereas physical symptoms, such as hot flushes and night sweats showed only a minor degree of association with past PMS.

Associated symptoms such as depression, mood changes, weight gain, fatigue and insomnia are not characteristic of the menopause, but do genuinely appear more frequent at this time. From our experience this seems to be more to do with dietary and lifestyle inadequacies than falling oestrogen levels. Changing your diet and lifestyle at the time of the menopause we have found to be as effective as the changes suggested for

PMS sufferers. Magnesium and the essential fatty acids appear to be important in the normal functioning of the ovaries. Making sure that there is an adequate supply of these and other nutrients may help ease the passage of menopausal symptoms.

Interestingly, in the Orient menopausal symptoms are less of a problem than they are in the West, and this has been attributed to the effects on hormone metabolism of a diet low in fat, high in fibre, soya, protein (which contains naturally occurring oestrogens) phyto-oesterols, and plenty of fresh fruit and vegetables.

Thinning of the bones leading to osteoporosis is particularly likely to accelerate around menopause with the loss of protective oestrogen. Calcium and exercise can limit this process and a specialized supplement rich in calcium, magnesium and multi-vitamins, Gynovite, is helpful at this time and supplements of Efacal (evening primrose oil, marine fish oil and calcium) provided by Efamol have been shown to reduce the amount of calcium lost through the urine and to increase the uptake of calcium across the gut wall. Many women are unable to take hormone replacement therapy (HRT), either for medical reasons, or because they experience side-effects. For example, it is thought that one-third of women on HRT experience symptoms of PMS, and of course they continue to have a monthly bleed. For the last eight years the WNAS has been providing a programme for women experiencing menopausal symptoms with a great deal of success.

Hormone replacement therapy has become very popular in the US and is being greeted with much enthusiasm in many quarters of the UK. It can be taken in the form of pills similar to oral contraceptives, as an implant inserted under the skin or as a patch applied to the skin of the abdomen or buttock. Some women swear by it, but two-thirds of women who try it come off within the first nine months because of side-effects or dissatisfaction, so there has to be a natural alternative.

In my experience over the last 10 years, finding the right diet to suit your body, taking specific nutritional supplements in the short term and moderate regular exercise can only serve to improve your general well-being. Once you have learned what your body requires, not only do you stand a good chance of overcoming your symptoms, but you will be far more likely to improve your quality of life, and improve your chances of avoiding the illnesses that can occur later in life, like heart disease, mental illness, or cancer.

22

MEN WHO NO
LONGER SUFFER

I didn't feel that the book would be complete without giving a voice to the men in our lives. I have concentrated so far on how women suffer with PMS. But it's not just women who suffer, let's face it, the men are very definitely on the receiving end! Women who have supportive partners have a far easier time on the programme than those whose partners refuse to acknowledge the condition and instead of being understanding, just simply fight back and turn off.

I have had the good fortune to hear from many men who were deeply concerned about the welfare of their women, once they understood that PMS was a real condition, which would respond to treatment. Last Christmas one husband took the telephone from his wife's hand and said I'd given him the best Christmas present he'd ever had. We often get told by men that 'they got back the girl they married'.

I think it's important for women to stand back and examine some of the viewpoints, in retrospect, of men who have lived with PMS sufferers before, during and after their nutritional programme. I'm happy to say they can mostly look back and laugh, probably with relief, for the storm is over.

Tom Moor, Jane's husband, is relieved to say that he got back the girl he married.

'Jane was very irritable, she couldn't hold a conversation without snapping. I couldn't touch her for two weeks before her periods as her breasts were so sore and tender. She rarely wanted to go out and would make excuses to stay at home. When she had PMS she changed from being very happy-go-lucky to being bitchy, irritable and tired.

When she was pre-menstrual I used to keep out of her way. I still showed her that I loved her and waited patiently for her one good week each month.

We were hoping for an early menopause.

The nutritional programme has made a tremendous difference to our lives. We are able to lead a normal life again. My wife laughs and jokes and she is popular at work.

My advice to other men is to seek help as it is available. Once their partner is on a nutritional programme, help her to persevere, as it will pay dividends in the long run. I feel that more education for men is necessary, more widespread information directed at couples. I, like most men, was totally baffled as to what the cause of the problem was.'

Don, June Garson's husband couldn't imagine what the consequences might have been had she not received help.

'Generally speaking I am a calm, tolerant person. I tried to make allowances, but I didn't understand the problem. It was like living with a "time bomb" not knowing when it was going to go off! June was permanently "uptight" and tearful pre-menstrually. She was unable to cope with life or deal with the children rationally.

Once on the nutritional programme an immediate improvement was noticeable. Her new-found state of mind and feeling of well-being turned the clock back to the time when we met, prior to our children being born. She reverted back personality-wise to the girl I fell for. I no longer dread the time of the month.

My advice to other men is as follows:

Be totally committed to discussing the subject in detail with your partner, read extensively on the subject and INSIST on her seeking help, not only for her sake, but for the rest of the family. Ignorance of the subject is the major hurdle to overcome.

I found your literature and your "cure" very interesting as I employ 150 people, many of them women. As a result of my experience with my wife I was able to realize that a staff problem affecting many employees was due to the PMS of a particular female employee. I have been able to discuss her problem sympathetically and we hope to solve the unrest in the office, as on my recommendation she has written to you for your help.'

Nadine's boyfriend felt that the biggest change for him was that he no longer had to duck to avoid the flying saucepans!

'Nadine's hysterical and often violent acts of throwing objects did cause anger, but more usefully, it improved my reaction time and my catching abilities no end!'

Life was difficult to cope with for Nadine. There were times of great frustration when new remedies for PMS failed to work. Since introducing the nutritional programme into her life, the quality of life for Nadine and her partner has increased enormously.

'I think the key to coping with PMS is to be patient and caring. If her irritability makes you irritable, then feel it, but don't show it. If her hysteria is frightening then allow yourself to be afraid, but be bigger than your fear, and calm her down. Be practical, do the cooking or take over the task she is finding difficult to cope with. Give up your time because you can bet she's feeling worse than you've ever done, and deserves your understanding and a shoulder to lean on. Tell her you love her and reassure her, and most of all, mean it.'

This bittersweet excerpt is from a letter written by the husband of one of our patients:

'I am Dodd, a roofing contractor with eight children and a wife with severe PMS symptoms. She was a complete Jekyll and Hyde character when her PMS struck.

Knowing what divorce can do to a family, I had to have the patience of Job with Eleanor. But after violent attacks (both on myself and the children), outrageous outbursts, locking herself into hotel rooms, insults, screams of rage, alienation from reality, a suicide attempt, and jealous behaviour I had had it. Bearing in mind that for most of the month she was warm, affectionate and everything a wife should be.

The worst of it all was after an attack when the illness had left her and she would creep back to me. Then I had to play the part of the caring husband again.

How can you expect a young couple with two children to come to terms with this terrible PMS problem when there is nowhere to go, nobody to see them? PMS is a dreadful affliction. It is self-destructive, life-threatening and family-life threatening. When I was a child, I would go to see a horror film and on it would be a pit of snakes – provided you did not disturb them they left you alone but woe betide you if you disturbed them. It was the same with Eleanor if she stuck to the diet or went on a binge.

Women are such beautiful creatures, advanced both mentally and physically from the male. More adaptable, stronger, philosophical, and yet they have to cope with some of the most awful female problems. Is this the price a woman has to pay for her beauty?

Eleanor is now cured of her PMS symptoms. I know she is cured and the WNAS has been responsible. The reason (after trying everything else) I know they have hit the nail on the head is because if complacency sets in and she starts pinching sweets, eating curries and drinking, I can guarantee by the end of her monthly cycle she will be going through agony. I am eternally grateful.'

His advice to other men is as follows:

1. A woman has to realize that she has a problem and that it is not everybody else around her that is wrong, but herself.

2. If and when she realizes this, she is 49 per cent there.

3. She has to get the husband to realize (buy him a dummy to suck; he will need it to bite hard on). You are then 98 per cent there.

4. The last 2 per cent is really just the beginning. When it has been realized, you still have an awful long way to go. But it is like everything else in life, you do not get owt for nowt. This now is when you really have to work hard. It is just like any other illness – if left untreated, it just gets worse.

Isn't that great? What wonderful understanding! The common factor for most men who are supportive, seems to be that they were educated on the subject of PMS. When they don't understand what's going on, they obviously find it more difficult to be supportive in the long term, which is quite understandable.

On behalf of PMS sufferers I would like to thank the supportive men of the world for being willing to share the problem. With more education, communication and understanding in the future on the subject of PMS, far fewer lives will be needlessly disrupted.

PART FOUR

APPENDICES

1 DICTIONARY OF TERMS

Abbreviations used

g = gram, mg = milligram (100 mg = 1 g), mcg = microgram (100 mcg = 1 mg),
iu = international unit, kj = kilojoule

ADRENAL GLANDS. The adrenal glands are two small glands situated at the top of the kidneys. They produce several different hormones, most of which are steroid hormones. Hormones from the adrenal glands influence the metabolism of sugar, salt and water and several other functions.

ALDACTONE. This is a diuretic drug which helps fluid retention. It inhibits the action of aldosterone, a hormone from the adrenal glands. It is also known as spironolactone.

ALDOSTERONE. This is a steroid hormone produced by the adrenal glands which is involved in salt and water balance. When it is produced in excess it causes the body to hold water and sodium salt.

ALLERGY. An unusual and unexpected sensitivity to a particular substance which causes an adverse reaction. Foods, chemicals and environmental pollutants are common irritants and they may cause a whole range of symptoms including headaches, abdominal bloating and discomfort, skin rashes, eczema and asthma.

AMENORRHOEA. A complete absence of periods.

AMINO ACIDS. Chains of building blocks which combine together to form the proteins that make living things. There are some 20 or more amino acids, some of which are essential and some non-essential.

ANTI-DEPRESSANTS. These are drugs used to suppress symptoms of depression.

BROMOCRIPTINE. A powerful drug, used to suppress the hormone prolactin. Further details of this can be found in Chapter 12, on conventional remedies. It is occasionally used in the treatment of PMS.

CARBOHYDRATES. Carbohydrates are the main source of calories (kjs) in almost all diets. *Complex carbohydrates* are essential nutrients and occur in the form of fruits, vegetables, pulses and grains. They are important energy-giving foods. There are two sorts of complex carbohydrates: the first are digestible, such as the starches, and the second are not digestible and are more commonly known as 'fibre'.

Refined carbohydrates. These consist of foods that have been processed and refined. White or brown sugar and white flour have, in the process of refining, had many of the vitamins and minerals present in the original plant removed. Further details on this may be found in Chapter 11.

CERVIX. The neck of the womb which projects downwards into the vagina.

CORPUS LUTEUM. Literally, a little yellow gland or body. It is the part of the ovary that remains after the egg has left. It produces two hormones, oestrogen and progesterone, during the second half of the menstrual cycle.

DAY 1 OF CYCLE. The first day of the menstrual bleeding, the day the period arrives, is the first day of the menstrual cycle.

DEFICIENCY. A lack of an essential substance, e.g. a vitamin.

DIURETICS. Drugs which cause an increased production of urine by the kidneys. They are used to treat fluid retention.

DOPAMINE. Dopamine is a brain chemical affecting mood. It has a sedating effect.

DYSMENORRHOEA. This is a term used to describe pain occurring during periods.

ENDOCRINE GLANDS. Glands that secrete hormones and regulate other organs in the body. The thyroid and the pituitary glands are endocrine glands.

ENDOMETRIOSIS. A condition in which the lining of the uterus begins to grow outside the uterus in the abdominal cavity. It is usually a painful condition and can be a cause of infertility.

ENDORPHINS. Hormones from the pituitary gland and fluid in the spine which are believed to help control moods, behaviour and part of the workings of the pituitary gland itself. They may also have an effect on how sugar is used in the body, and on other amounts of hormones released from the pituitary gland and the ovaries. If this is so, the production of oestrogen and progesterone could be affected by endorphins.

ESSENTIAL FATTY ACIDS. One of the essential groups of foods which we need to eat to remain healthy. These are essential fats that are necessary for normal cell structure and body function. There are two: linoleic and linolenic acids. They are called 'essential' as they cannot be made by the body but have to be eaten in the diet.

FALLOPIAN TUBES. A pair of slender tubes through which the egg passes on its way from the ovary to the uterus. Fertilization occurs in the Fallopian tubes. Very rarely the egg remains in the tube and grows: this is called an ectopic pregnancy, and is a medical emergency accompanied by severe abdominal pain.

FOLLICLE. A small sac in the ovary containing an egg (ovum). After release of the egg at mid-cycle the follicle becomes a corpus luteum.

FOLLICLE STIMULATING HORMONE (FSH). A hormone of the pituitary gland which stimulates the growth of the follicles in the ovaries.

FOLLICULAR PHASE. The first half of the menstrual cycle when an egg is growing in the ovary. The egg is surrounded by cells which produce the hormone oestrogen and which thus prepares the uterus for conception. The egg and surrounding cells are called a follicle.

GLUCOSE. A form of sugar, found in the diet or released by the liver into the bloodstream, which is then used by the brain for energy. This is the only source of energy usable by the brain.

GRAAFIAN FOLLICLE. A mature egg which is surrounded by a bag of fluid within the ovary.

HORMONES. Substances formed chiefly in the endocrine glands, which then enter the bloodstream and control the activity of an organ or body function. Adrenaline and insulin are hormones, as are oestrogen and progesterone.

HYPERHYDRATION – TOO MUCH WATER PRESENT. This is a term used to describe water retention in the body.

HYPOGLYCAEMIA – LOW BLOOD SUGAR. This is a condition in which there is a deficiency of glucose in the bloodstream, often caused by an excess of insulin or a lack of food. As glucose is required for normal brain function, mental disturbance can occur as can other symptoms: headaches, weakness, faintness, irritability, palpitations, mood swings, sweating and hunger. One of the commonest contributing factors is an excess of refined carbohydrates in the diet.

HYPOTHALAMUS. The region of the brain controlling temperature, hunger, thirst and the hormones produced by the pituitary gland.

HYSTERECTOMY. A surgical procedure to remove the womb and the Fallopian tubes. Sometimes one or more ovaries are also removed.

LUTEAL PHASE. The time after the egg has left the follicle in the ovary, and the follicle then becomes a gland known as the corpus luteum. The corpus luteum produces progesterone.

LUTEINIZING HORMONE (LH). The pituitary hormone which fosters the development of the corpus luteum.

MENORRHAGIA. An excessive loss of blood during each period.

MENSES. The discharge of blood and tissue lining from the uterus, which occurs approximately every four weeks between puberty and the menopause.

MENSTRUAL CYCLE. The monthly cycle involving the pituitary gland, ovaries and uterus in which an egg is produced ready for conception to take place. In each cycle an egg in the ovary is released and the lining of the womb develops ready for conception and implantation of the fertilized egg. If this does not occur, the lining of the womb is shed and a period occurs.

MENSTRUAL SYMPTOMATOLOGY DIARY. A chart which is a daily record of all symptoms that occur throughout the menstrual cycle.

METABOLISM. The process by which the body maintains life. It is the cycle of nutrients being broken down to produce energy, which is then used by the body to build up new cells and tissues, provide heat, growth, and physical activity. The metabolic rate tends to vary from person to person, depending on their age, sex and lifestyle.

MITTELSCHMERZ. Pain associated with ovulation. It occurs usually at the time of ovulation, about halfway through the cycle. Translated, it means 'middle pain'.

NUTRITION. The British Society for Nutritional Medicine's definition is 'the sum of the processes involved in taking nutrients, assimilating and utilizing them'. In other words, the quality of the diet and the ability of your body to utilize the individual nutrients and so maintain health.

OESTROGEN. A steroid hormone which is produced in large quantities by the ovaries, and in smaller amounts by the adrenal glands. It is responsible for the development of breasts and other sexual characteristics at puberty. Oestrogen is also responsible for the production of fertile cervical mucus, the opening of the cervix, and building up of blood in the lining of the uterus, preparing for a fertilized egg.

OVARIES. A pair of glands situated on either side of the uterus, in which eggs and sex hormones, including oestrogen, are produced.

OVULATION. The release of the ripe egg (ovum) from the ovary. The two ovaries ovulate alternately every month. Occasionally, the two ovaries ovulate simultaneously, in which case the result may be twins.

OVUM. The egg which is released from the ovary at the time of ovulation.

PALPITATIONS. The heart beating too fast and sometimes irregularly.

PITUITARY GLAND. A small gland situated at the base of the brain, which produces many hormones, among which are those which stimulate the ovary and the thyroid.

PRE-MENSTRUAL. A term used to describe the time before the arrival of a period.

PRE-MENSTRUAL SYNDROME. This is the name given to a collection of mental and physical symptoms which manifest themselves before the onset of a period.

PRE-MENSTRUAL TENSION. This was the name first given to the symptoms detected before a period in 1931 by Dr Frank. Now the correct name is Pre-Menstrual Syndrome. However, many women still prefer to call the condition PMT – Pre-Menstrual Tension.

PROGESTERONE. A hormone secreted by the corpus luteum of the ovary during the second half of the menstrual cycle. Some studies have shown that a deficiency in progesterone may be responsible for some PMS symptoms. Progesterone is an important hormone during pregnancy.

PROGESTOGENS. A group of synthetic hormones, with actions similar to progesterone.

PROLACTIN. The hormone secreted by the pituitary gland which is involved in milk production. It is also known to affect water and mineral balance in the body, and in some women may play a part in the changes pre-menstrually.

PROSTAGLANDINS. Hormone-like substances found in almost every cell in the body, which are necessary for the normal function of involuntary muscles, including the heart, the uterus, blood vessels, the lungs and the intestines.

Prostaglandins are sometimes regarded as health controllers, as they seem to play an important part in the controlling of many essential functions in the body. They do not come directly from the diet, but are made in the body itself. Because of this, the body relies on a

271

good diet in order to produce prostaglandins. The special substances that the body needs to make these hormones are called essential fatty acids.

SEROTONIN. A brain chemical that influences mood.

STEROIDS. Substances which have a particular chemical structure in common. All the sex hormones, such as oestrogen, progesterone, etc are steroids.

THYROID GLAND. A gland situated in the neck, which produces the hormone thyroxine. The thyroid gland regulates metabolism.

TRANQUILLIZERS. A group of drugs which artificially sedate the body. They may be useful in the short term, but in the long term they can have addictive qualities.

UTERUS (WOMB). A sac-like organ which is located in the abdomen of a woman, and designed to hold and nourish a growing child from conception until birth.

VAGINA. The passage that leads from the uterus to the external genital organs.

2 FOOD ADDITIVES

There are many types of food additives. Most of them are denoted by a number prefixed by E. The E stands for EEC, as the European Community Regulations state that, since 1 January 1986, all foods containing additives, except for flavourings, must have an E number, or the actual name, in the list of ingredients. Some food additives are natural, vegetable-derived compounds, or even vitamins, and are perfectly harmless. However, these are not used frequently. The following additives can be associated with the exacerbation of certain medical problems:

Azo-dyes E102, E104, E107, E110, E122, E123, E124, E128, E131, E132, E133, E142, E151, E154, E155, E180

Benzoates E210–E219

Sulphur dioxide and sulphites E220–E227

Nitrites and nitrates E249–E252

Proprionic acid and propionates E280–E283

Anti-oxidants, BHA & BHT E320 and E321

Monosodium glutamate (MSG) and related compounds E621–E623

Many food allergy associations now give details of suppliers of foods suitable for people who suffer from allergies. Some of these are mentioned on page 276. Many supermarkets will now provide lists of their products which are free from additives, milk, wheat, eggs, etc. For those who wish to request further details, it is suggested that you contact the customer relations department of the appropriate supermarket chain.

The Ministry of Agriculture, Fisheries and Food has produced a booklet explaining what the 'E' numbers mean. There is also the excellent book 'E for Additives' by Maurice Hanssen, which is readily available. An organization called 'Foresight', The Association for the Promotion of Pre-Conceptual Care, have produced a handbag-sized booklet based on the information from the book 'E for Additives'. They have marked additive numbers with a colour code, red for danger, and they specify precisely why, orange for those additives on which conflicting reports still exist, and green for those about which there are no known side-effects. This booklet is immensely valuable as it takes the confusion out of shopping. You will find the Foresight address in Appendix 5 should you wish to obtain a copy.

3 NUTRITIONAL SUPPLEMENT SUPPLIERS

1.	Efamol	Boots, chemists, healthfood shops and Nutritional Health (mail order)*
2.	Femvite	Nutritional Health (mail order)*.
3.	Linusit Gold	Healthfood shops.
4.	Magnesium Hydroxide Mixture	Boots and other chemists.
5.	Optivite	Nutritional Health (mail order)*
6.	Natural Vitamin E	Healthfood shops and Nutritional Health (mail order)*
7.	Sugar Factor/Normoglycaemia	Nutritional Health (mail order)*

*Mail Order Address
Please send a stamped addressed envelope for the catalogue.
Nutritional Health Ltd
PO Box 926
Lewes, East Sussex
BN7 2QL

Australia

NNFA (National Nutrition Foods Association)
PO Box 84, Westmead, NSW 2145. Tel: 02 633 9913
The NNFA have lists of all supplement stockists and retailers in Australia, if you have any difficulties in obtaining supplements.

New Zealand

NNFA (National Nutrition Foods Association)
c/o PO Box 820062, Auckland, New Zealand.
Again the NNFA have lists of all supplement stockists and retailers in New Zealand, if you have any difficulties in obtaining supplements.

4 RECOMMENDED READING LIST

NOTE
UK, USA and A denotes the following books are available in Great Britain, United States and Australia. Out of print titles may be available via libraries.

GENERAL HEALTH

Pure, White and Deadly by Professor John Yudkin (a book about sugar) price £9.95 (published by Viking). **UK A**
Coming off Tranquillizers by Dr Susan Trickett (Thorsons). **UK USA A** (Lothian Publishing Co).
The Migraine Revolution – The New Drug-free Solution by Dr John Mansfield (Thorsons). **UK USA A** (Lothian Publishing Co).
Understanding Cystitis by Angela Kilmartin (Arrow Books). **UK A**
The Book of Massage (Ebury Press). **UK**
Do-it-yourself Shiatsu by W. Ohashi (Unwin Hyman). **Out of print UK**
Candida Albicans: Could Yeast Be Your Problem? by Leon Chaitow (Thorsons). **UK USA A** (Lothian Publishing Co).
Candida Albicans by Gill Jacobs (Optima). **UK USA A**
Nutritional Medicine by Dr Stephen Davies and Dr Alan Stewart (Pan Books). **UK A**
The Y Plan Countdown (Hamlyn). **UK**
Bone Boosters – Natural Ways to Beat Osteoporosis by Diana Moran and Helen Franks (Boxtree Limited). **UK**
The Migraine Handbook by Jenny Lewis (Vermilion). **UK A**
The Book of Yoga, Sivananda Yoga Centre (Ebury Press). **UK A**

DIET

The Vitality Diet by Maryon Stewart and Dr Alan Stewart (Optima). **UK A**
Good Food Gluten-Free by Hilda Cherry Hills (Keats Publishing Inc.). **USA**
The Wheat and Gluten Free Cookbook by Joan Noble (Vermilion). **UK A**
The New Why You Don't Need Meat by Peter Cox (Bloomsbury). **UK A**
Beat Sugar Craving by Maryon Stewart (Vermilion). **UK A**
The Allergy Diet by Elizabeth Workman SRD, Dr John Hunter and Dr Virginia Alun Jones (Vermilion). **UK USA**
The Candida Albicans Yeast-Free Cook Book by Pat Connolly and Associates of the Price Pottenger Nutrition Foundation (Keats Publishing Inc). **UK USA**
The Cranks Recipe Book by David Canter, Hay Canter and Daphne Swann (Grafton). **UK**
The Food Intolerance Diet by Elizabeth Workman SRD, Dr Virginia Alun Jones and Dr John Hunter (Optima). **Out of print UK USA**
The New Raw Energy by Leslie and Susannah Kenton (Vermilion). **UK A** (Doubleday Publishing Co).
The Reluctant Vegetarian by Simon Hope (William Heinemann). **UK**
The Salt-Free Diet Book by Dr Graham McGregor (Optima). **Out of print UK USA**

Gourmet Vegetarian Cooking by Rose Elliot (Thorsons). **UK A**
Healthy Cooking from Tesco Stores. **UK**
Food Allergy and Intolerance by Jonathan Brostoff and Linda Gamlin (Bloomsbury).
UK A
The Gluten-free and Wheat-free Bumper Bake Book by Rita Greer (Bunterbird Ltd). **UK**

STRESS

Self-Help for your Nerves by Dr Clair Weekes (Thorsons). **UK USA** (Hawthorn
Publishing Co).
Stress and Relaxation Self-Help Techniques for Everyone by Jane Madders (Optima). **UK
USA A**
Lyn Marshall's Instant Stress Cure (Vermilion). **UK A**

GENERAL

How to Stop Smoking and Stay Stopped for Good by Gillian Riley (Vermilion). **UK A**
Getting Sober and Loving It by Joan and Derek Taylor (Vermilion). **Out of print UK A**
The National Childbirth Book of Breast Feeding by Mary Smale (Vermilion). **UK**
Tired all the Time by Dr Alan Stewart (Vermilion). **UK USA A**
Memory Power by Ursula Markham (Vermilion). **UK A**
Aromatherapy by Gill Martin (Vermilion). **UK USA A**
Acupuncture by Dr Michael Nightingale (Vermilion). **UK USA A**
Alternative Health Osteopathy by Stephen Sandler (Optima). **UK USA A**
Beat the Menopause Without HRT by Maryon Stewart (Headline). **UK**
Every Woman's Heath Guide by Maryon Stewart and Dr Alan Stewart (Headline) **UK**
Healthy Parents, Healthy Baby by Maryon Stewart (Headline)

5 USEFUL ADDRESSES

UK

Accept Clinic
724 Fulham Road, London SW6 5SE.   Tel: 0171 371 7477

Action against Allergy
PO Box 278, Twickenham TW1 42Q

Action on Phobias
c/o Shandy Mathias, 8-9 The Avenue, Eastbourne, East Sussex. Letters only enclosing sae.

Alcoholics Anonymous (AA)
General Services Office, PO Box 1, Stonebow House, Stonebow, York YO1 2NJ.
Tel: 01904 644026

Amarant Trust
11-13 Charter House Buildings, London EC1M 7AN.   Tel: 01293 41300

Anglo-European Collee of Chiropractitioners
13-15 Parkwood Road, Bournemouth BH5 2DF.   Tel: 01202 436 200

Anorexia & Bulimia Care
Tottenham Women's Health Centre, 15 Fenhurst Gate, Aughton, Ormskirk,
Lancs L39 5ED.   Tel: 01695 422479

Association for Post Natal Illness
25 Jerdan Place, London SW6 1BE.   Tel: 0171 386 0868

ASH (Action on Smoking and Health)
Devon House, 12-15 Dartmouth Street, London SW1H 9BL.   Tel: 0171 314 1360

Asset (Exercise Association)
4 Angel Gate, City Road, London EC1V 2PT.   Tel: 0171 278 0811

British Acupuncture Register and Directory
34 Alderney Street, London SW1V 4UE   Tel: 0171 834 1012

British Association for Counselling
1 Regent Place, Rugby, Warwickshire CV21 2PJ.   Tel: 01788 578328 (info)

British College of Naturopathy and Osteopathy
6 Netherhall Gardens, London NW3 5RL.   Tel: 0171 435 6464

The British Homeopathic Association
27a Devonshire Street, London W1N 1RJ.   Tel: 0171 935 2163

British Hypnotherapy Association
67 Upper Berkeley Street, London W1H 7DH.   Tel: 0171 723 4443

British Osteopathic Association Clinic
8-10 Boston Place, London.   Tel: 0171 262 1128

British School of Osteopathy
Administration and Clinics, 1-4 Suffolk Street, London SW1Y 4HG.   Tel: 0171 930
9254

British Pregnancy Advisory Service
Austy Manor, Wootton Warren, Solihull, West Midlands B95 6BX.   Tel: 01564 793225

British Society for Allergy and Clinical Immunology
66 Western Park, Thames Ditton, Surrey K17 O16. Fax: 0181 398 2766

British Wheel of Yoga
1 Hamilton Place, Boston Road, Sleaford, Lincolnshire NG34 7ES.   Tel: 01529 306851

Bristol Cancer Help Centre
Grove House, Cornwallis Grove, Clifton, Bristol BS8 4PG

Brooks Advisory Clinic
165 Grays Inn Road, London WC1X 8UD.   Tel: 0171 713 9000

Coeliac Society
PO Box 220, High Wycombe, Bucks HP11 2HY.   Tel: 01494 37278

Chiropractic Patients Association
8 Centre One, Lysander Way, Old Sarum Park, Salisbury, Wiltshire SP4 6BU.
Tel: 01722 416027

The Council for Acupuncture
206-208 Latimer Road, London W10 2RE.   Tel: 0181 964 0222

Depression Alliance
PO Box 1022, London SE1 7QB.   Tel: 0171 721 7672

The European School of Osteopathy
104 Tonbridge Road, Maidstone, Kent ME16 8SL.   Tel: 01622 671558

Eating Disorders Association
Sackville Place, 44 Magdalen Street, Norwich, Norfolk NR3 1JU.   Tel: 01603 621414

Foresight Association for the Promotion of Preconceptual Care
28 The Paddock, Godalming, Surrey GU7 1XD.   Tel: 01483 427839

The Faculty of Homoeopathy
The Royal Homoeopathic Hospital, Hannemann House, 2 Powis Place, Gt Ormond Street,
London WC1N 3HT

Food Watch International
Butts Pond Industrial Estate, Sturminster Newton, Dorset DT10 1AZ.   Tel: 01258 73356

Friends of the Earth
26-28 Underwood Street, London N1 7JQ.   Tel: 0171 490 1555

The Henry Doubleday Research Association
Ryton Gardens, National Centre for Organic Gardening, Ryton on Dunsmore, Coventry
CV8 3LG.   Tel: 01203 303517

Homoeopathic Development Foundation
19a Cavendish Square, London W1M 9AD.   Tel: 0171 629 3205

International Federation of Aromatherapists
4 Eastmearn Road, West Dulwich, London SE21 8HA

London Food Commission
3rd Floor, 5-11 Worship Street, London EC2A 3BH.   Tel: 0171 628 7774

Marriage Guidance Council
76A New Cavendish Street, London W1M 7LB. Tel: 0171 580 1087

Medau Society
8b Robson House, East Street, Epsom, Surrey KT17 1HH.   Tel: 013727 29056

Migraine Trust
45 Great Ormond Street, London WC1 3HZ.   Tel: 0171 278 2676

The ME Association
Stanhope Place, High Street, Stanford-le-Hope, Essex SS17 0HA

National Asthma Campaign
Providence House, Providence Place, London N1 0NT

National Council for One-Parent Families
255 Kentish Town Road, London NW5 2LX.   Tel: 0171 267 1361

The National Endometriosis Association
Suite 50, Westminster Palace Gardens, 1-7 Artillery Road, London SW1R 1RL.
Tel: 0171 222 2781

The National Institute of Medical Herbalists
56 Longbrook Street, Exeter EX4 6AN.   Tel: 01392 426022

National Society for Research into Allergy
PO Box 45, Hinkley, Leicestershire LE10 1JY.   Tel: 01455 303517

Patients' Association
8 Guildford Street, London WC1N 1DT.   Tel: 0171 242 3460

Positively Women
347-349 City Road, London EC1V 1LR.   Tel: 0171 713 0222

Release
388 Old Street, London EC1V 9LT.   Tel: 0171 729 9904

The Samaritans
10 The Grove, Slough SL1 1QP.   Tel: 01753 532713

School of Phytotherapy (Herbal Medicine)
Bucksteep Manor, Bodle Street Green, Nr. Hailsham BN27 4RJ.   Tel: 01323 833812/4

The Shiatsu Society
31 Pullman Lane, Godalming, Surrey GU7 1XY.   Tel: 01483 860 771

The Soil Association
86-88 Colston Street, Bristol BS1 5BB.   Tel: 01272 290661

The Sports Council
16 Upper Woburn Place, London WC1H 0QP.   Tel: 0171 388 1277

Tranx Release (Northampton)
Anita Gordon, 81 St Giles Street, Northampton NN1 1JF.   Tel: 01604 22121

Trax (UK) Ltd.
National Tranquillizer Advice Centre, Registered Office, 25a Masons Avenue, Wealdstone,
Harrow, Middlesex HA3 5AH.   Tel: (client line) 0181 427 2065 (24 hour answering
service 0181 427 2827)

UK College for Complementary Healthcare Studies
St Charles Hospital, Exmoor Street, London W10 6D2.   Tel: 0181 9641206

Vegan Society
Donald Watson House, 7 Battle Road, St. Leonards-on-Sea, East Sussex TN3Y 7AA

Vegetarian Society
Parkdale, Dunham Road, Altrincham, Cheshire WA14 4QG.   Tel: 0161 928 0793

Women's Health
52 Featherstone Street, London EC1Y 8RT.   Tel: 0171 251 6580

The Women's Nutritional Advisory Service
PO Box 268, Lewes, East Sussex BN7 2QN.   Tel: 01273 487366

Women's Therapy Centre
6-9 Manor Gardens, London N7 6LA.   Tel: 0171 263 6200

YMCA
112 Great Russell Street, London WC1B 3NQ.   Tel: 0171 637 8131

AUSTRALIA

Women's Health Statewide
64 Pennington Terrace, Nth Adelaide SA 5006.   Tel: (08) 8267 5366

Women's Health Advisory Service
155 Eaglecreek Road, Werombi NSW 2570.   Tel: 046 531 445

The Evening Primrose Oil Information Service
9/1 Vuko Place, Warriewood NSW 2102.   Tel: (02) 9970 8622 (Sydney).
Tel: 1800 064 953 (elsewhere in Australia)

Women's Infolink
280 Adelaide St, Brisbane QLD 4000.   Tel: (07) 3229 1580

Women's Information & Referral Exchange
247 Flinders Lane, Melbourne VIC 3000.   Tel: (03) 9654 6844

Women's Information Service
122 Kintore Ave, Adelaide SA 5000.   Tel: (08) 8223 1244

Tresillian Family Care Centre
2 Shaw St, Petersham NSW 2049.   Tel: (02) 9568 3633

Nutritional Foods Association of Australia
PO Box 104, Deakin West ACT 2600.   Tel: (06) 260 4022

Blackmores Advisory Limited
23 Roseberry Street, Balgowlah, NSW 2093.   Tel: (02) 9949 3177.

Royal Society for the Welfare of Mothers and Babies
2 Shaw Street, Petersham, NSW 2049.   Tel: (02) 568 3633.

Childbirth Education Association of Victoria
21 Greensborough Centre, 25 Main Street, Greensborough, Victoria 3088.

Liverpool Women's Health Centre
26 Bathurst Street, Liverpool NSW 2170.   Tel: (02) 9601 3555.

Adelaide Women's Community Health
64 Pennington Terrace, Nth Adelaide SA 5006.   Tel: (08) 267 5366.

PMT Relief Clinic
Suite 6, 32 Kensington Road, Rose Park, South Australia 5067.   Tel: (08) 364 2760.

Efamol (Australia)
9/1 Vuko Place, Warriewood NSW 2102.   Tel: (02) 9970 8622

NEW ZEALAND

Papakura Women's Centre
4 Opaneke Road, Papakura, Auckland.   Tel: (09) 299 9466.

Whakatane Women's Collective
PO Box 3049, Ohope.   Tel: (Whakatane) 076 24757.

Health Alternative for Women
Room 101, Cranmer Centre, PO Box 884, Christchurch.   Tel: (03) 796 970.

Women's Health Collective
63 Ponsonby Road, Ponsonby, Auckland.   Tel: (09) 764 506.

West Auckland Women's Centre
111 McLeod Road, Te Atatu, Auckland.   Tel: (09) 8366 381.

Tauranga Women's Centre
PO Box 368, Tauranga.   Tel: (075) 783 530.

The Alice Bush Family Planning Clinic
214 Karangahape Road, Auckland.   Tel: (09) 775 049.

Family Planning Clinic
Arts Centre, 301 Montreal Street, Christchurch.   Tel: (03) 790 514.

Efamol (New Zealand)
PO Box 33, 118 Takapura, Auckland 1332 NZ.   Tel: (09) 415 8477

USA AND CANADA

National Institute of Nutrition
1565 Carling Avenue, #400, Ottawa, Ontario K12 8R1.

The American Academy of Environmental Medicine
PO Box 16106, Denver, Colorado 80216.

Optimox Inc
PO Box 3378, Torrance, California 90510–3378.   Tel: (800) 223 1601.

6 CHARTS AND DIARIES

SYMPTOMS	WEEK AFTER PERIOD (Fill in 3 days after period)				WEEK BEFORE PERIOD (Fill in 2-3 days before period)			
	None	Mild	Moderate	Severe	None	Mild	Moderate	Severe
PMS - A								
Nervous Tension								
Mood Swings								
Irritability								
Anxiety								
PMS - H								
*Weight Gain								
Swelling of Extremities								
Breast Tenderness								
Abdominal Bloating								
PMS - C								
Headache								
Craving for Sweets								
Increased Appetite								
Heart Pounding								
Fatigue								
Dizziness or Fainting								
PMS - D								
Depression								
Forgetfulness								
Crying								
Confusion								
Insomnia								
OTHER SYMPTOMS								
Loss of Sexual Interest								
Disorientation								
Clumsiness								
Tremors/Shakes								
Thoughts of Suicide								
Agoraphobia								
Increased Physical Activity								
Heavy/Aching Legs								
Generalized Aches								
Bad Breath								
Sensitivity to Music/Light								
Excessive Thirst								

Do you have any other PRE-MENSTRUAL SYMPTOMS
not listed opposite? Use this page to make a note of these.
'Weight Gain' in the chart opposite refers to the amount
you put on before your period.

MENSTRUAL SYMPTOMATOLOGY DIARY

Month: _____

GRADING OF MENSES

0–none	3–heavy
1–slight	4–heavy and
2–moderate	clots

GRADING OF SYMPTOMS (COMPLAINTS)

0–none
1–mild-present but does not interfere with activities
2–moderate-present and interferes with activities but not disabling
3–severe-disabling. Unable to function.

Day of cycle																													
Date																													
Period																													

PMS - A

Nervous tension																													
Mood swings																													
Irritability																													
Anxiety																													

PMS - H

Weight gain																													
Swelling of extremities																													
Breast tenderness																													
Abdominal bloating																													

PMS - C

Headache																													
Craving for sweets																													
Increased appetite																													
Heart pounding																													
Fatigue																													
Dizziness or faintness																													

PMS - D

Depression																													
Forgetfulness																													
Crying																													
Confusion																													
Insomnia																													

PAIN

Cramps (low abdominal)																													
Backache																													
General aches/pains																													
Frequency of sex (tick day)																													
Enjoyment of sex (0-10)																													

NOTES:

MENSTRUAL SYMPTOMATOLOGY DIARY

Month: _____

GRADING OF MENSES

0–none	3–heavy
1–slight	4–heavy and
2–moderate	clots

GRADING OF SYMPTOMS (COMPLAINTS)

0–none
1–mild-present but does not interfere with activities
2–moderate-present and interferes with activities but not disabling
3–severe-disabling. Unable to function.

Day of cycle																															
Date																															
Period																															

PMS - A

Nervous tension																															
Mood swings																															
Irritability																															
Anxiety																															

PMS - H

Weight gain																															
Swelling of extremities																															
Breast tenderness																															
Abdominal bloating																															

PMS - C

Headache																															
Craving for sweets																															
Increased appetite																															
Heart pounding																															
Fatigue																															
Dizziness or faintness																															

PMS - D

Depression																															
Forgetfulness																															
Crying																															
Confusion																															
Insomnia																															

PAIN

Cramps (low abdominal)																															
Backache																															
General aches/pains																															
Frequency of sex (tick day)																															
Enjoyment of sex (0-10)																															

NOTES:

7 REFERENCES

Below is a list of some of the more important references relating to studies detailed in this edition of the book. The WNAS has endeavoured over the years to keep details of most of the important studies on the causation and treatment of PMS. A copy of these references and other information on PMS can be obtained from the WNAS by sending £3 in postage stamps to The Women's Nutritional Advisory Service, PO Box 268, Lewes, Sussex BN7 2QN.

Chapter 1

1. Green R., Dalton K. The Pre-Menstrual Syndrome. British Medical Journal. May 9, 1953. P1007–1014.
2. Abraham G.E. Nutrition and the Pre-Menstrual Tension Syndromes. Journal of Applied Nutrition. 36:103–124. 1984.
3. Morton J.H., Additon H., Addison R.G., Hunt L., Sullivan J.J. A clinical study of Pre-Menstrual Tension. A.M.J.Obstet.Gynecol. 55:1182–1191. 1953.

Chapter 2

1. Abraham G.E. Management of the Pre-Menstrual Tension Syndromes: Rationale for a Nutritional Approach. In: A Year in Nutritional Medicine, Second Edition 1986. Ed. by Bland J. Keats Publishing, Inc. New Canaan, Connecticut: 125–166. 1986.
2. Munday M.R., Brush M.G., Taylor R.W. Correlation between Progesterone, Oestradiol and Aldosterone Levels in the Pre-Menstrual Syndrome. Clinical Endocrinology. 14:1–9. 1981.
3. Watts J.F.F., Butt W.P., Logan Edwards R., Holder G. Hormonal Studies in Women with Pre-Menstrual Tension. British Journal of Obstetrics and Gynaecology. 92:247–255. 1985.
4. Dalton M.E. Sex Hormone-Binding Globulin Concentrations in Women with Severe Pre-Menstrual Syndrome. Post-Graduate Medical Journal. 57:560–561. 1981.

Chapter 3

1. Moos R.H. Typology of Menstrual Cycle Symptoms. American Journal of Obstet.Gynec. 103:390–402. 1969.

Chapter 4

1. Dalton K. Pre-Menstrual Syndrome and Progesterone Therapy. Second Edition. William Heinemann Medical Books Limited London. 1984.
2. Hargrove J.T., Abraham G.E. The Incidence of Pre-Menstrual Tension in a Gynaecologic Clinic. The Journal of Reproductive Medicine. 27:721–724. 1982.
3. Hargrove J.T., Abraham G.E. The Ubiquitousness of Pre-Menstrual Tension in a Gynaecologic Practice. The Journal of Reproductive Medicine. 28:435–437. 1983.

Chapter 5

1. Yudkin J. Pure, White and Deadly. Viking Press. London. 1986.
2. Royal College of General Practitioners. Alcohol – A Balanced View. Report from General Practice 24. RCGP London. 1986.
3. Drug Abuse Briefing. Institute for the Study of Drug Dependents. London. 1986.

4. Abraham G.E. Nutrition and the Pre-Menstrual Tension Syndromes. Journal of Applied Nutrition. 36:103–124. 1984.
5. Ashton C.H. Caffeine and Health. The British Medical Journal. 295:1293–4. 1987.

Chapter 6

1. Boyle C.A. et al. Caffeine Consumption and Fibrocystic Breast Disease: A Case-Control Epidemiologic Study. JNCI. 72:1015–1019. 1984.
2. O'Brien P.M.S, Selby C., Symonds E.N. Progesterone, Fluid and Electrolytes in Pre-Menstrual Syndrome. The British Medical Journal. 10 May 1980: 1161–1163.
3. MacGregor G.A. et al. Is 'Idiopathic' Oedema Idiopathic. The Lancet 1:397–400. 1979.
4. O'Brien P.M.S., Selby C., Symonds E.M. Progesterone, Fluid and Electrolytes in Pre-Menstrual Syndrome. The British Medical Journal. 280:1161–3. 1980.

Chapter 7

1. Yudkin J. Pure, White and Deadly. Viking Press. London. 1986.
2. Morton J.H., Additon H., Addison R.G., Hunt L., Sullivan J.J. A clinical study of Pre-Menstrual Tension. A.M.J.Obstet.Gynecol. 55:1182–1191. 1953.

Chapter 8

1. Abraham G.E. Nutrition and the Pre-Menstrual Tension Syndromes. Journal of Applied Nutrition. 36:103-124. 1984.
2. Dalton K. Pre-Menstrual Syndrome and Progesterone Therapy. Second Edition. William Heinemann Medical Books Limited London. 1984.

Chapter 9

1. Dalton K. Pre-Menstrual Syndrome and Progesterone Therapy. Second Edition. William Heinemann Medical Books Limited London. 1984.

Chapter 10

1. Pre-Menstrual Syndrome – Proceedings for Workshop held at the Royal College of Obstetricians and Gynaecologists. London, 2nd December 1982. Ed. Taylor. R.W. Medical News – Tribune Limited. London. 1983.
2. Sampson J.A. Pre-Menstrual Syndrome: A Double-Blind Control Trial of Progesterone and Placebo. British Journal of Psychiatry. 135:209–215. 1979.
3. Dennerstein L., et al. Progesterone and the Pre-Menstrual Syndrome: A Double-Blind Cross Over Trial. British Medical Journal. 290:1617–1621. 1985.
4. Magos A., Studd J. Progesterone and the Pre-Menstrual Syndrome: A Double-Blind Cross Over Trial. British Medical Journal. 291:213–214. 1985.
5. O'Brien P.M.S. The Pre-Menstrual Syndrome: A Review of the Present Status of Therapy. Drugs 24:140–151. 1982.

Chapter 11

1. Modern Nutrition in Health and Disease. Ed: Goodhart R.S., Shils M.E. Sixth edition Lea and Febiter, Philadelphia. 1980.
2. Nutritional Medicine. Davies S., Stewart A. Pan Books London. 1987.
3. Lewis J., Buss D.H. Trace Nutrients 5. Minerals and Vitamins in the British Household Food Supply. British Journal of Nutrition. 60:413–424. 1988.
4. Spring J.A., Robertson J., Buss D.H. British Journal of Nutrition. 41:487–493. 1979.

5. Gregory J., Foster K., Tyler H. and Wiseman M. The Dietary and Nutritional Survey of British Adults. HMSO. London 1990.
6. Committee on Medical Aspects of Food Policy. Dietary Reference Values for Food Energy and Nutrients for the United Kingdom. HMSO. London 1991.

Chapter 12

1. Piesse J.W. Nutrition Factors in the Pre-Menstrual Syndrome. International Clinical Nutrition Review. 4:54–81. 1984.
2. Hargrove J.T., Abraham G.E. Effect of Vitamin B6 on Infertility in Women with Pre-Menstrual Syndrome. Infertility 2:315–322. 1979.
3. Abraham G.E., Hargrove J.T. The Effect of Vitamin B6 on Pre-Menstrual Symptomatology in Women with Pre-Menstrual Syndrome: A Double-Blind Cross Over Study. Infertility. 3:155–165. 1980.
4. Gunn A.D.G. Vitamin B6 and the Pre-Menstrual Syndrome. In Vitamins-Nutrients as Therapeutic Agents. Ed: Hanck A., Hornig D. Hans Huber Publishers. Bern. 1985. P213–224.
5. Stokes J., Mendels J. Pyridoxine and Pre-Menstrual Tension. The Lancet 1:1177–1178. 1972.
6. Abraham G.E. Magnesium Deficiency in Pre-Menstrual Tension. Magnesium Bulletin 1:68–73. 1982.
7. Abraham G.E., Lubran M.M. Serum and Red Cell Magnesium levels in patients with Pre-Menstrual Tension. The American Journal of Clinical Nutrition. 34:2364–2366. 1981.
8. Sherwood R.A., Rocks B.F., Stewart A., Saxton R.S. Magnesium in the Pre-Menstrual Syndrome. Ann. Clin. Biochem. 23:667–670. 1986.
9. Pre-Menstrual Tension: An Invitation a Symposium. Ed. Abraham G.E. Journal of Reproductive Medicine. 28:7 & 8:433–538. 1983.
10. Fushs N., Hakim M., Abraham G.E. The Effect of a Nutritional Supplement, Optivite, for Women with Pre-Menstrual Tension Syndromes. 1. Effect of Blood Chemistry and Serum Steroid levels during the mid-luteal phase. The Journal of Applied Nutrition. 37:1–11. 1986.
11. Chakmakjian Z.H., Higgins C.E., Abraham G.E. The Effect of a Nutritional Supplement, Optivite, for Women, on Pre-Menstrual Tension Syndromes: 2. The effect of Symptomatology, using a Double-Blind Cross-Over Design. The Journal of Applied Nutrition. 37:12–17. 1986.
12. London, R.S. et al. The Effect of Alpha-Tocopherol on Pre-Menstrual Symptomatology: A Double-Blind Study. Journal of the American College of Nutrition. 2:115–122. 1983.
13. London, R.S. et al. The Effect of Alpha-Tocopherol on Pre-Menstrual Symptomatology: A Double-Blind Study 2. Endocrine correlates. Journal of the American College of Nutrition. 3:351–356. 1984.
14. O'Brien P.M.S. Pre-Menstrual Syndrome. Blackwell Scientific Publications, Oxford, 1987.
15. Stewart A. A Rational Approach to Treating Pre-Menstrual Syndrome. WNAS publication, 1989.
16. Stewart A. Clinical and Biochemical Effects of Nutritional Supplementation on the Pre-Menstrual Syndrome. The Journal of Reproductive Medicine. 32:435–441. 1987.
17. Boyd E.M.F. et al. The effect of a low-fat, high complex-carbohydrate diet on symptoms of cyclical mastopathy. The Lancet. 2:128–132. 1988.
18. Freeman E., Rickels K., Sondheimer S.J. and Polansky M. Ineffectiveness of Progesterone Suppository Treatment for Pre-Menstrual Syndrome. Journal of the American Medical Association. 264:349–53. 1990.
19. Kleijnen J., ter Riet G. and Knipschild P. Vitamin B6 in the Treatment of Pre-Menstrual Syndrome: A Review. British Journal of Obstetrics and Gynaecology.

97:847–852. 1990.
20. London R.S., Bradley L. and Chiamori N.Y. Effect of a Nutritional Supplement on Pre-Menstrual Symptomatology in Women with Pre-Menstrual Syndrome: A Double-Blind Longitudinal Study. Journal of the American College of Nutrition. 10:494–499. 1991.

Chapter 14

1. Yudkin J. Pure, White and Deadly. Viking Press, London. 1986.
2. Royal College of General Practitioners. Alcohol – A Balanced View. Report from General Practice, 24. RCGP. London 1986.
3. Health Education Council. That's The Limit – Booklet. HEC, 78 New Oxford Street, London EC1A 1AH.
4. Nutritional Medicine by Dr Stephen Davies and Dr Alan Stewart. Pan Books. 1987.
5. Which? Troubled Waters, Which? November 1986. P494–497.
6. Spring J.A., Robertson J., Buss D.H. Trace Nutrients 3. Magnesium, Copper, Zinc, Vitamin B6, Vitamin B12 and Folic Acid in the British Household Food Supply. Br.J.Nutr. 41:487–493. 1979.
7. Victor B.S., Greden J.F., and Lubetsky, M. Somatic Manifestations of Caffeinism. J.Clin Psychiat. 42:185–8. 1981.
8. Disler P.B. et al. The Effects of Tea on Iron Absorption. Gut 18:193–200. 1975.
9. Tonkin S.Y. Vitamins and Oral Contraceptives. In Vitamins in Human Biology in Medicine. Ed: Briggs M.H. CRC Press, Boca Raton, Florida. P29–64. 1981.
10. Walters A.H., Fletcher J.R., Law S.J. Nitrate in Vegetables: Estimation by HPLC. Nutrition and Health. 4:141–149. 1986.
11. Mount J.L. The Food and Health of Western Man. Charles Knight & Co Ltd, London. 1975.
12. The Booker Health Report – A Survey of Vitamin and Mineral Intakes within Certain Population Groups. Booker Health Foods. 1986.

Chapter 19

1. Chuong C.J., Coulam C.B., Kao P.C., Bergstalh J., Go V.L.W. Neuropeptide levels in Pre-Menstrual Syndrome. Fertility and Sterility. 44:760–765. 1985.
2. Prior J.C., Vigna Y. and Alojada N. Conditioning Exercise Decreases Pre-Menstrual Symptoms. European Journal of Applied Physiology. 55:349–355. 1986.

INDEX

abdomen:
  bloating, 13, 17, 37-46, 179, 189
  curl-over exercises, 242
  pain, 15
Abraham, Dr Guy, 2, 16, 121, 133,
    170, 203
aches, generalized, 13, 18, 143
acne, 13, 135, 149, 199, 204
acupressure, 246-8
acupuncture, 246, 251, 257
additives, food, 98, 108, 133, 272
adrenal glands, 10, 11
adrenaline, 47, 229
advice lines, 301
aerobic exercise, 234, 235
ageing, 16
aggression, 21
agoraphobia, 13, 18, 72-7, 230
alcohol, 48, 108, 148, 177, 229
  and clumsiness, 69
  consumption levels, 97-8, 99
  effects of, 110-11
  vitamin and mineral deficiencies,
    102, 135, 136
allergies, 96, 119, 200, 229-30
  to grains, 179-89
  to yeast, 189-94
almond:
  almond macaroons, 226-7
  lemon and almond cake, 227-8
aluminium, 107, 108
amino acids, 10, 100, 126
anaemia, 48, 134, 135, 149, 204, 252,
    256
ankles, swollen, 13
anorexia nervosa, 256
antacids, 108
anti-anxiety dugs, 118
antibiotics 98, 105, 119, 207
anti-depressants, 99, 117-18, 207, 260
anxiety, 13, 17, 19, 20, 118, 121, 233,
    246-7
appetite, increased, 17, 47
apples:
  apple and cinnamon cake, 226

stuffed baked apples, 223
apricots:
  dried fruit conserve, 210
aromatherapy oils, 231
ascorbic acid see vitamin C
asthma, 13, 108
Ativan, 99
autogenic training, 231
avocados:
  avocado and yoghurt dressing, 214
  fresh avocado and tomato soup,
    211-12

back, tension-releasing exercises,
    240-1
backache, 13, 230, 233, 235, 244-6
bad breath, 13, 18
baking powder, 181
bananas:
  banana cream, 223-4
  ginger bananas, 224
barley, 179, 184
batter, grain-free, 181
beanshoot salad, 212
Beatty, Cheryl, 71-2
benzodiazepenes, 99
beta-carotene, 129, 259
beta-endorphin, 234
beverages, 152, 153, 186
  see also alcohol; coffee; tea
biscuits:
  almond macaroons, 226-7
  grain-free, 182, 184
  potato shortbread, 226
Biskind, Dr, 2
blackcurrant seed oil, 123
bloating, 13, 17, 37-46, 179, 189, 190
blood sugar levels, 47-8, 198
boils, 13
bones see osteoporosis
borage oil, 123
brain:
  control of hormones, 10-11
  food cravings, 47
  glucose and, 128

menstrual cycle, 7
bran, 133
bread:
  buckwheat and rice bread, 225
  grain-free, 179-80, 184
  potato and rice bread, 225
breadcrumbs, grain-free, 181
breakfast:
  menus, 150-1, 185
  recipes, 209-10
breakfast cereals, 181
breast-feeding, 131, 133, 256, 258
breasts, 205
  cancer, 97, 132
  lumps, 15
  swollen, 13
  tenderness, 13, 15, 17, 37-46, 116,
    117, 118, 123, 127, 200, 203
breathing, 20, 236, 239
broccoli soup, 211
Bromocriptine, 117
Brown, Gail, 53-6, 91
buckwheat and rice bread, 225
bulgar and nut salad, 213
Burton, Natasha, 22-6, 92
Buspirone, 118

caffeine, 19-20, 48, 109, 110, 175
cakes:
  apple and cinnamon cake, 226
  carrot cake, 223
  coconut pyramids, 227
  fruity cakes, 224
  ginger cake, 227
  grain-free, 181, 184
  lemon and almond cake, 227-8
calcium, 107, 108, 111, 132-3, 137-8,
  160-1, 175, 260, 262
cancer, 95-6, 97, 98, 107, 129, 132
Candida albicans, 119, 190
carbohydrates, 38, 127-8, 136
  cravings, 17, 47-56
carbon dioxide, hyperventilation, 20
cardiovascular disease, 95
cardiovascular training, 235

carotene, 96
carrot cake, 223
cars, driving ability, 91-2, 143
case histories:
  Cheryl Beatty, 49-53, 71-2
  Claire, viii-ix, 43-6, 56
  Clare, 92
  Frankie Ferguson, 89-90
  Gail Brown, 53-6, 91
  Geraldine Ellis, 139
  Grace Edwards, 63-5
  Hazel, 73-7
  Iona, 87-8
  Jane Moor, 263-4
  Janet, 65-8
  Judy Harrington, 82-4
  Julie Masters, 40-3
  June Garson, 264
  Marcia, 81-2
  Marilyn, 60-3
  Maureen, 32-6, 90-1
  Melanie, 194-8
  Natasha Burton, 22-6, 92
  Pauline, 68
  Rebecca Harley, 140-1
  Sally, 193-4
  Sandra Patterson, 139-40
  Sarah, 27-32
  Sonia, 191-3
cereals:
  nutritional content, 155-62
  pesticides, 98
  sensitivity to, 179-89
cervix, 6, 7, 9
charts, 163, 165-9, 281-4
chicken, 105-6
  chicken soup, 212
  stuffing for roast, 222
chilli and peanut dressing, 214
chocolate, 47, 48, 49, 52, 53, 56, 63,
  97, 175
cholesterol, 106, 127, 128, 131
chromium, 103, 132, 136, 149, 150,
  198
cigarettes *see* smoking

clumsiness, 13, 18, 69-70, 234
coconut pyramids, 227
cod liver oil, 132, 259
coffee, 19-20, 38, 48, 69, 97, 109, 112, 135, 136, 148, 172, 175, 200
  substitutes, 109, 148, 152, 186
colourful lentils, 221-2
Committee on the Medical Aspects of Food, 101
confusion, 13, 18, 143
constipation, 13, 110, 122, 128, 179, 184
contraceptive pill see oral contraceptive pill
convenience foods, 133, 134
cooking methods, 104
copper, 103, 107, 108, 132
corn, 181, 184
corpus luteum, 9
cramps, 13, 231, 233
cranial osteopathy, 244-5, 251
cravings, 13, 17, 47-56, 136, 197, 198-9, 205
crime, 77-9
crying, 13, 18, 230, 259
cucumber and orange salad, 213
curl-overs, 242
custard, egg, 224-5
Cyclogest, 114
cystitis, 13, 189, 190

dairy produce, 132, 148, 175, 200
Dalton, Dr Katharina, 2-3, 13, 58, 60, 77
Danazol, 116, 253
dandelion coffee, 109, 175
dandruff, 200, 204, 205
daydreaming, 230
Department of Health, 101, 121, 258, 259
depression, 13, 117, 179
  acupressure, 246-7
  exercise and, 233, 234
  menopause, 261

oral contraceptives and, 99
PMS D (depression), 18, 57-68, 139, 149, 169, 205
  post-natal, 73, 259-60
  stress and, 230
  yeast sensitivity and, 189, 190
desserts, recipes, 222-5
diabetes, 128
diaries, 161-3, 281-4
diarrhoea, 13, 124, 179, 230
diet and nutrition, 16, 18, 126-9
  additives, 98, 108, 133, 272
  allergies, 96, 119, 179-94, 200, 229-30
  ancestors' diet, 96, 105
  carbohydrates, 38, 127-8
  cholesterol, 106, 127, 128, 131
  choosing a nutritional plan, 147-63
  cooking methods, 104
  effects on menstrual cycle, 10-11
  essential fatty acids, 127, 199-200, 251, 258-9
  fats, 19, 97, 105-6, 127, 163
  fibre, 19, 128
  habits, 111-12
  nitrates, 98, 107
  nutritional content, 155-63
  and oestrogen levels, 19
  organic produce, 105, 107, 150
  pesticides, 98
  phosphorus, 97, 132-3, 176
  polyunsaturated fats, 105, 127, 163
  processed food, 104, 176, 229
  proteins, 126-7, 178
  salt content, 37-8, 97
  saturated fats, 97, 106
  and stress, 229
  sugar content, 97, 106
  tailor-made nutritional programme, 164-207
  treatment of PMS, 120-4
  twentieth-century changes, 97-8
  vegetarian and vegan, 131, 135, 178
  water, 128-9

dinner:
  menus, 151, 153, 186, 187
  recipes, 215-22
disorientation, 13, 18
distress, 229
diuretics, 118, 134, 135
dizziness, 13, 17, 48
Doxycycline, 119
dressings *see* salad dressings
dried fruit:
  dried fruit compote and yoghurt,
    222
  dried fruit conserve, 210
driving ability, 91-2, 143
drugs, 76-9, 99, 205, 207, 257
  treatment of PMS, 117-19
dydrogesterone, 115

eating disorders, 117
eczema, 13, 108, 123, 127, 135, 199,
    200, 204, 205
Edwards, Grace, 63-5
Efamol, 127, 139, 200, 203, 205, 206,
    262
eggs, 253
  egg custard 224-5
  nutritional content, 155-8, 160-2
  Spanish omelette, 216
eggs (ova), 6-9, 256, 260
Ellis, Geraldine, 139
emotional stress, 11
endometriosis, 115, 116, 250
endometrium, 6
endurance, muscular, 235
epilepsy, 124, 207
essential fatty acids, 127, 137-8, 163,
    199-200, 251, 258-9, 262
evening primrose oil, 120, 123, 124,
    127, 137-40, 200, 203, 205-7
exercise, 11, 16, 57, 148-9, 231, 232,
    233-43, 251, 262
eye problems, 204
eye strain, 230

facial hair, 15

fainting, 13, 17, 48
Fallopian tubes, 7, 250, 260
fatigue, 13, 17, 48, 179, 199, 261
fats, in diet, 19, 97, 105-6, 127, 163
Femvite, 124, 203, 205, 206
Ferguson, Frankie, 89-90
fertilization, 7
fertilizers, nitrate, 98, 107
fibre, dietary, 19, 128, 251
fibroids, 250, 252-3
fish, 105, 148
  fish oils, 137-8, 148, 163, 251
  grilled (broiled) sardines, 215
  mackerel with herbs (in foil), 217-
    18
  nutritional content, 155-63
  steamed fish with garlic, spring
    onions and ginger, 219
  stuffed mackerel in foil, 218
flatulence *see* wind
flours, grain-free, 180-2
fluid retention, 37-8, 97, 118, 129,
    134, 246
Fluoxetine, 117
folic acid, 101, 131, 158, 258
follicles, 7-9
food *see* diet and nutrition
Food and Drug Administration
    (USA), 101
food additives, 98, 108, 133, 272
food cravings, 13, 17, 39, 47-56, 117,
    197-9, 205
food sensitivity, 201
  to grains, 179-89
  to yeast, 189-94
fool, rhubarb, 223
forgetfulness, 13
fragrant lamb, 200
Frank, Dr Robert T., 2, 12
Freeman, Dr, 114
fructose, 127
fruit, 98, 100, 107
  dried fruit compote and yoghurt,
    222
  dried fruit conserve, 210

fruit jelly, 222
fruity cakes, 224
hot fruity breakfast, 210
nutritional content, 155-62
see also apples; bananas etc

gallstones, 128
gamma-linolenic acid, 123
Garson, June and Don, 264
ginger:
    ginger bananas, 224
    ginger cake, 227
glucose, 47, 127, 128
goals, 231
goulash, vegetarian, 218
grains, sensitivity to, 179-89
grapefruit and orange salad, 213
green bean and sweetcorn salad, 213-14
green leafy vegetables, 177, 253
Greene, Dr Raymond, 3
growth hormones, 98
Gynovite, 262

hair, facial, 15
hair problems, 199, 204
Harley, Rebecca, 140-1
Harrington, Judy, 82-7
Harris, Dr, 2
hayfever, 13
headaches, 13, 15, 17, 194-8, 233, 239
    acupressure, 247
    caffeine and, 20
    cravings and, 48
    oral contraceptives and, 99, 115
    osteopathy, 244-5
    pain-killers, 118
    stress and, 230-1
heart:
    exercise, 235
    heart disease, 95, 97, 106, 128
    palpitations, 20, 47
    pounding, 13, 17, 48
heat therapy, 251-2

herbal teas, 110, 148, 152, 175, 186
hives, 13
honey, 176, 190
hormones:
    causes of PMS, 3, 16, 19
    cholesterol and, 127
    effect on mood and behaviour, 9, 10
    and exercise, 234
    hormone replacement therapy (HRT), 115-16, 262
    menstrual cycyle, 7, 9
    treatment of PMS, 113-17, 207
    see also oestrogen; progesterone
hostility, 13
hyperactivity, 108
hyperventilation, 20
hypoglycaemia, 47
hypothalamus, 10-11

implants, hormonal, 115, 116, 262
infertility, 199
insomnia, 13, 18, 20, 68, 118, 205, 230, 247, 259
iron, 102-3, 132, 149, 178, 260
    deficiency, 48, 134-5, , 137-8, 139, 199, 251, 252-3
    sources of, 161
    tea and, 110
    vitamin C and, 131
irritability, 13, 17, 19, 30-1, 233, 259
irritable bowel syndrome, 40, 230
Israel, Dr, 2
IUDs (coils), 199, 253

jelly, fruit, 222
joints:
    problems, 13, 233
    suppleness, 235-6
'junk food', 147-8, 176, 229

Kelly, Donna, 78
kidneys, 128-9
Kimberly-Clark, 89

lactose, 127
lamb:
    fragrant lamb, 200
    lamb paprika, 200
lead pollution, 107, 108
legs, aching or restless, 13, 18
leisure activities, 232
lemon and almond cake, 227-8
lentils:
    colourful lentils, 221-2
    lentil and vegetable soup, 210-11
libido, 70-2, 199
light sensitivity, 13, 18
linoleic acid, 127
linolenic acid, 127
linseed, 184, 200, 205
lithium, 119
liver, functions, 126, 127, 128
liver (in diet), 253, 259
    liver with orange, 221
Lovell, Debra, 78
Lubran, Dr, 121
lunch:
    menus, 151, 152, 185, 187
    recipes, 215-22
lungs, exercise, 235

macaroons, almond, 226-7
McCance, Dr, 2
mackerel:
    mackerel with herbs (in foil), 217
    stuffed mackerel in foil, 218
magnesium, 11, 38, 107, 132
    alcohol and, 111
    and anxiety, 19
    deficiency, 102, 133-4, 137-8, 140
    and depression, 57
    diuretics and, 118
    and fatigue, 48
    and the menopause, 262
    and painful periods, 250-2
    ans post-natal depression, 260
    side-effects, 124
    sources of, 161-2, 177
    treatment with, 121-2

and vitamin B6, 130
manganese, 103
mango delight, 228
marijuana, 48
massage, 231
Masters, Julie, 40-3
meat, 148, 150
    fat content, 105
    nutritional content, 155-62
    pesticides in, 98
meditation, 231
mefenamic acid, 118, 250
men, living with PMS sufferers, 263-6
menopause, 5, 116, 246, 252, 261-2
menstrual cycle, 5-11, 256
mental illness, 96, 229
menus, 150-4, 185-9
mercury, 107
metabolism, 125-6, 233
migraine, 13, 40, 99, 115, 118, 194,
    198, 230, 245, 246
milk, 98
minerals, 100, 132-6
    deficiencies, 136-8, 203-4
    supplements, 202-6, 253, 257
    toxic, 107-8
Mogadon, 99
mood swings, 13, 17, 19, 20, 230,
    233, 259
Moor, Jane and Tom, 263-4
Morris, Nadine, 264-5
mouth:
    cracking at corners, 189, 199, 204
    ulcers, 13, 179, 204
mucus, cervical, 6, 7
muesli, 209-10
multi-vitamins, 107, 122-3, 203, 253,
    259
muscles, 125, 127
    endurance, 235
    relaxation, 231
    strength, 235

nail problems, 199, 204
Naltrexone, 119

neck, tension-releasing exercises, 239-40
nerve damage, 124
nerves, 125
nervous tension, 13, 17, 19, 20-1, 205, 230, 233
nicotinamide *see* vitamin B3
nicotinic acid *see* vitamin B3
nipples, discharges, 15
nitrates, 98, 107
noise sensitivity, 13
noodles:
    rice, 180-1
    snow peas with tiger prawns, 219-20
norethisterone, 115
nutrition *see* diet and nutrition
nuts, 148
    bulgar and nut salad, 213
    nut roast, 221
    nutritional content, 155-63
    nutty parsnip soup, 211

oats, 179, 184
obesity, 128
oestrogen, 121
    causes of PMS, 2, 17, 19
    effect on mood and behaviour, 9
    menopause, 261
    menstrual cycle, 7, 9
    the Pill, 99, 115
    and suicidal feelings, 59
    treatment of PMS, 115-16
oil and fruit dressing, 215
oils, 160
    aromatherapy, 231
    fish, 137-8, 148, 163, 251
    vegetable, 148
    vitamin E content, 160
omelette, Spanish, 216
Optivite, 89, 121-4, 203, 205, 206
oral contraceptive pill, 16, 19, 99-100, 115, 135, 139, 191, 200, 250, 253
oranges:

grapefruit and orange salad, 213
liver with orange, 221
orange and cucumber salad, 213
organic produce, 105, 107, 150
osteopathy, 244-5
osteoporosis, 11, 117, 175, 233, 256, 262
ovaries, 250, 257, 260
    false menopause, 117
    hormone production, 7-9, 10, 11, 114
    magnesium and, 57
    menopause, 261, 262
    menstrual cycyle, 6-9
overweight, 39, 57, 141
ovulation, 6-9
Owen, Nicola, 78

pain:
    abdominal, 15
    period, 14, 115, 118, 205, 247-8, 249-52
pain-killers, 118, 250
palpitations, 20, 47, 205
pancakes:
    grain-free, 181
    wholewheat, 209
panic attacks, 19
parsnip soup, nutty, 211
pasta, grain-free, 180-1, 184
patches, hormonal, 116, 262
Patterson, Sandra, 139-40
peanut and chilli dressing, 214
pelvic tilt, 238, 241-2
peppers:
    Spanish omelette, 216
    stuffed peppers, 216
periods:
    heavy, 15, 115, 116, 135, 149, 199, 252-3
    irregular, 15, 246, 256-7
    painful, 14, 115, 118, 205, 247-8, 249-52
pessaries, progesterone, 114
pesticides, 98

phosphates, 133
phosphorus, 97, 132-3, 176
phytic acid, 133
the Pill *see* oral contraceptive pill
pituitary gland, 7, 10-11, 117, 140,
    257, 261
PMT (supplement), 206
pollution, 16, 98, 107-8, 112
polysaccharides, 128
polyunsaturated fats, 105, 127, 163
post-natal depression, 73, 259-60
posture, 235, 238, 239, 245
potassium, 38, 118, 132, 134
potatoes:
    potato and rice bread, 225
    potato shortbread, 226
prawns, snow peas with, 219-20
Pre-Menstrual Syndrome (PMS):
    causal factors, 16
    drug treatment, 117-19
    hormonal treatment, 113-17
    incidence, 95-7
    nutritional treatment, 120-4
    PMS A (anxiety), 17, 19-36, 149,
        150, 166-9, 205, 233
    PMS C (carbohydrate craving), 17,
        47-56, 149, 150, 169, 205
    PMS D (depression), 18, 57-68,
        139, 149, 169, 205
    PMS H (hydration), 17, 37-46,
        149, 169, 205
    sub-groups, 18
    symptoms, 12, 13, 16-18
Pre-Menstrual Tension (PMT), 12
pregnancy, 9, 131, 133-4, 246, 256-9
preservatives, 98, 108
processed food, 104, 176, 229
progestagens, 115
progesterone, 116, 203
    causes of PMS, 2, 3, 17
    effect on mood and behaviour, 9
    menstrual cycle, 7, 9
    and post-natal depression, 259
    and sterilization, 261
    treatment of PMS, 114-15

prolactin, 117
proteins, 126-7, 178
Prozac, 117
psoriasis, 135
pulses, nutritional content, 155-62
pyridoxine *see* vitamin B6

raising agents, 181
raw food, 177-8
recipes, 208-28
relationships, 16, 80-7, 111, 143
relaxation, 231-2, 233, 234, 236, 242-
    3, 251
religion, 1
restlessness, 13, 230
retinol, 129, 259
Reynolds, Anna, 78
rhubarb fool, 223
riboflavin *see* vitamin B2
rice:
    buckwheat and rice bread, 225
    potato and rice bread, 225
    rice noodles, 180-1
running, 235
rye, 179, 184

salad dressings:
    avocado and yoghurt, 214
    creamy tomato, 215
    oil and fruit, 215
    peanut and chilli, 214
    yoghurt herb, 214-15
salads, 148, 177
    beanshoot, 212
    bulgar and nut, 213
    grapefruit and orange, 213
    green bean and sweetcorn, 213-14
    orange and cucumber, 213
    Waldorf, 212-13
salt, 37-8, 97, 118, 122, 128-9, 134,
    148, 175-6, 200
sardines, grilled (broiled), 215
saturated fats, 97
schizophrenia, 60
sedatives, 118

selenium, 103, 132, 162
sensitivity *see* food sensitivity
serotonin, 117
sex drive, 13, 18, 65, 70-2
sex hormones *see* oestrogen;
   progesterone
Shiatsu, 246-8
shortbread, potato, 226
shoulders, tension-releasing exercises,
   239-40
skin problems, 108, 135, 149, 200,
   204, 205
sleep *see* insomnia
sleeping tablets, 99, 118, 207
smoking, 48, 69, 98, 106, 136, 148,
   149, 177, 200
snacks, 151-2, 182, 185-6, 189, 257
snow peas with tiger prawns, 219-20
sodium, 132, 134
   see also salt
soups:
   avocado and tomato, 211-12
   broccoli, 211
   chicken, 212
   lentil and vegetable, 210-11
   nutty parsnip, 211
Spanish omelette, 216
sperm, 6, 7
Spironolactone, 118
sponge cakes, 181
stamina, 235
standing position, 238
starflower oil, 123
sterilization, 73, 260-1
stir-fry vegetables, 216-17
strength, 235
stress, 11, 16, 18, 96, 202, 229-32,
   256
Studd, John, 115
stuffing for roast chicken, 222
sucrose, 127, 128
sugar, 127-8, 130, 190
   consumption of, 38, 97, 106, 147-
   8, 176-7
   cravings, 13, 47-56, 136, 197, 198-
    9, 205
   and fluid retention, 38
suicidal feeling, 13, 18, 58-60, 259
supplements, 107, 202-6, 253, 257,
   273
suppleness, 235-6
sweetcorn and green bean salad, 213
sweets, recipes, 222-5
swimming, 233, 235
swollen extremities, 13, 17, 37-8
symptoms:
   of PMS, 12, 13, 16-18
   withdrawal, 172, 200

tea, 19-20, 38, 48, 69, 97, 103, 110,
   135, 136, 148, 172, 175, 200
teeth, signs of stress, 230
tension 230-1, 233, 236
   exercises to release, 239-43
   nervous tension, 13, 17, 19, 20-1,
    205, 230, 233
testosterone, 116
tetracycline, 207
thiamin *see* vitamin B1
thirst, 13, 18
thrush, 99, 119, 135, 139, 189, 190,
   193-4
thyroid gland, 10, 11, 48, 140, 260
tocopherol *see* vitamin E
tomatoes:
   avocado and tomato soup, 211-12
   creamy tomato dressing, 215
tongue, sore, 199, 204
toxic minerals, 107-8
trace elements, 103, 132
tranquillizers, 99, 207
tremors, 13, 18

urination, frequency of, 20
urine, 128
uterus, 133
   fibroids, 250, 252-3
   menstrual cycle, 6, 7, 9

vagina, 6

discharges, 15
infections, 119
soreness, 15
Valium, 76, 99
varicose veins, 128
vegan diet, 110, 178
vegetable oil, 148
vegetables, 148, 177
lentil and vegetable soup, 210-11
nutritional content, 155-62
stir-fry vegetables, 216-17
toxins, 98, 107
vegetarian goulash, 218
vitamins and minerals, 100
vegetarian diet, 105, 110, 131, 135, 178
vegetarian goulash, 218
violence, 21, 77-9, 143
vitamins, 10, 100, 129-32
deficiencies, 136-8, 203-4
multi-vitamins, 107, 122-3, 203, 253, 259
supplements, 202-6, 257, 273
vitamin A, 96, 129, 155, 259
vitamin B complex, 2, 19, 57, 101-2, 107, 124, 129-31, 198, 205, 229, 253, 256, 258, 260
vitamin B1 (thiamin), 111, 130, 137-8, 155
vitamin B2 (riboflavin), 108, 130, 155-6
vitamin B3 (nicotinic acid), 130, 156
vitamin B6 (pyridoxine), 11, 101, 111, 120-1, 123, 130-1, 137-8, 140, 149, 150, 156-7
vitamin B12 131, 157-8
vitamin C, 96, 107, 108, 110, 131, 135, 137-8, 149, 159, 253

vitamin D, 111, 127, 132, 259
vitamin E, 96, 121, 131-2, 149, 159-60, 205

Waldorf salad, 212
walking, 149, 230, 233
warming-up exercise, 238-9
water, 98, 107, 128-9, 133
water filters, 107-8
water retention, 37-8, 97, 118, 129, 134
water tablets, 118, 134, 135
weight gain, 13, 15, 17, 37-46
weight loss, 15, 39, 141, 256
wheat, 179, 184
wholefoods, 133, 135, 148
wholewheat, 179
wholewheat pancakes, 209
wind, 13, 178, 179, 189, 190
withdrawal symptoms, 172, 200
womb see uterus
work, 231-2
problems, 16
productivity and efficiency at, 87-91, 143

yeast sensitivity, 189-94, 198
yoga, 231, 251
yoghurt, 191
avocado and yoghurt dressing, 214
banana cream, 223-4
dried fruit compote and yoghurt, 222
yoghurt herb dressing, 214

zinc, 11, 103, 107, 110, 111, 132, 135-8, 140, 149, 162, 178, 199, 258

FURTHER HELP

If you would like information on the WNAS programme for pre-menstrual syndrome, or want to let me know about your success using the recommendations in this book, you can write to me at the following address.

If you require information, a large (A5) self-addressed envelope and four loose first-class stamps will guarantee you a reply; please state particularly that you are interested in receiving information on PMS, as we help women with all sorts of other conditions as well (see below).

Women's Nutritional Advisory Service
PO Box 268
Lewes
East Sussex BN7 2QN.
Tel: 01273 487366

ADVICE LINES
FROM THE WNAS

OVERCOME PMS NATURALLY	0839 556600
THE PMS DIET LINE	0839 556601
OVERCOME MENOPAUSE NATURALLY	0839 556602
THE MENOPAUSE DIET LINE	0839 556603
BEAT SUGAR CRAVING	0839 556604
THE VITALITY DIET LINE	0839 556605
OVERCOMING BREAST TENDERNESS	0839 556606
OVERCOME PERIOD PAINS NATURALLY	0839 556607
GET FIT FOR PREGNANCY AND BREASTFEEDING	0839 556608
SKIN, NAIL & HAIR SIGNS OF DEFICIENCY	0839 556609
IMPROVE LIBIDO NATURALLY	0839 556610
BEAT IRRITABLE BOWEL SYNDROME	0839 556611
OVERCOME FATIGUE	0839 556612
BEAT MIGRAINE NATURALLY	0839 556613
OVERCOME OVULATION PAIN	0839 556614
DIRECTORY	0839 556615

ALSO BY MARYON STEWART

If you have found this book helpful, you may be interested in her other titles published by Vermilion:

NO MORE IBS!   009 181593 2   £8.99

Available from all good bookshops or call our mail order hotline number on 01621 819596. Postage and packing is free.